OCCUPATIONAL
THERAPY
DISRUPTORS

What Global OT Practice Can Teach Us
About Innovation, Culture, and Community

SHEELA ROY IVLEV

Foreword by Juman Simaan

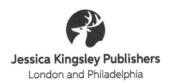

Jessica Kingsley Publishers
London and Philadelphia

First published in Great Britain in 2024 by Jessica Kingsley Publishers
An imprint of John Murray Press

1

Copyright © Sheela Roy Ivlev 2024

The right of Sheela Roy Ivlev to be identified as the Author of the Work has been
asserted by her in accordance with the Copyright, Designs and Patents Act 1988.

Foreword Copyright © Juman Simaan 2024

A CIP catalogue record for this title is available from the
British Library and the Library of Congress

ISBN 978 1 83997 665 0
eISBN 978 1 83997 666 7

Printed and bound in the United States by Integrated Books International

Jessica Kingsley Publishers' policy is to use papers that are natural, renewable
and recyclable products and made from wood grown in sustainable
forests. The logging and manufacturing processes are expected to conform
to the environmental regulations of the country of origin.

Jessica Kingsley Publishers
Carmelite House
50 Victoria Embankment
London EC4Y 0DZ

www.jkp.com

John Murray Press
Part of Hodder & Stoughton Limited
An Hachette UK Company

Occupational Therapy Disruptors

of related interest

Antiracist Occupational Therapy
Unsettling the Status Quo
Edited by Musharrat J. Ahmed-Landeryou
Foreword by Professor Elelwani Ramugondo
ISBN 978 1 83997 574 5
eISBN 978 1 83997 575 2

Roots and Rebellion
Personal Stories of Resisting Racism and Reclaiming Identity
Various Authors
Foreword by Dr Arun Verma
ISBN 978 1 83997 283 6
eISBN 978 1 83997 284 3

D.I.V.E.R.S.I.T.Y.
A Guide to Working with Diversity and Developing Cultural Sensitivity
Vivian Okeze-Tirado
ISBN 978 1 83997 631 5
eISBN 978 1 83997 632 2

Contents

FOREWORD BY JUMAN SIMAAN 7

ACKNOWLEDGEMENTS 15

Introduction 17

1. Uganda: Victor Alochi 19

2. Palestine: Moussa Abu Mostafa 33

3. Philippines: John Ray Lucas 45

4. Nepal: Dorothy Das Pariyar 55

5. Ghana: Ann Sena Fordie 65

6. United Kingdom: Musharrat Jabeen Ahmed-Landeryou . . 77

7. Aotearoa New Zealand: Isla Te Ara o Rehua Emery-
   Whittington 89

8. United States: Adam Cisroe Pearson 101

9. Brazil: Milena Franciely Rodrigues dos Santos 113

10. Thailand: Tunchanok Chunvirut 125

11. Iceland: Ósk Sigurdardottir 135

12. Botswana: Lady Gofaone Modise 145

13. Trinidad and Tobago: Khamara-Lani Tarradath 155

14. Bangladesh: Razia Sultana 167

15. Haiti: Ramona Joëlle Adrien 177

16. India: Sakshi Tickoo 189

ABOUT THE AUTHOR 201

Foreword

In *Notebook of a Return to the Native Land*, the Martiniquais poet Aimé Césaire explored the themes of self-identity and decolonization (1947/1984). Césaire wrote "no race holds a monopoly of beauty, of intelligence, of strength, and, there is a place for all at the Rendezvous of Victory." Césaire co-founded the Negritude movement that began among French-speaking African and Caribbean writers living in Paris as a protest against French colo- 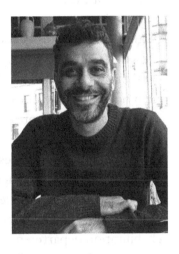 nial rule and the policy of assimilation. The Negritude movement became central to the struggle for Black liberation, such as the Civil Rights Movement in the United States of America (USA) and to the Black is Beautiful movement in North and South America. Césaire's poem speaks to me at this point in the history of occupational therapy and occupational science because it reaffirms my belief that there's no form of knowledge or practice that is superior to other forms, and that all means of knowing and doing should be welcomed and celebrated in what Boavuntura de Sosa de Santos described as the "ecologies of knowledges" (2014).

Occupational therapy's development, knowledge base, and practice was exclusive to white female practitioners when it first became a profession in the USA in 1917 (Black, 2002). It was only in 1943 that people of color were permitted to access occupational therapy programmes, but they needed to appear white-passing (Black, 2002). Almost 80 years later, not much progress had been achieved: for instance, 84 percent of occupational therapists in the USA still identify as white (American Occupational Therapy Association, 2020). The profession of occupational therapy was developed by and for middle- to upper-class white people using a dominant Eurocentric worldview. Consequently, occupational therapy has not addressed racial identity or disparity in developing assessments and interventions, or in monitoring outcomes for people of color, for example (Grenier, 2020).

It is about time we added to our shelves a book that amplifies crucial voices, experiences, and communities that we all need to be listening carefully to—a book that reaffirms our belief that there is more than one way of doing occupational therapy. This book is about envisioning a new world and seeking to transform minds and praxis, and it helps us to see our shared world differently.

Reading the stories presented in the book you're holding now, I was reminded of something I was recently told: "Our country desperately needs rehabilitation services, including physiotherapy, occupational therapy, and speech and language therapy." This was said by Abdullah, head of the rehabilitation department in the main public hospital in Freetown, the capital of Sierra Leone. He co-founded the first neuro rehabilitation department in his country, which currently employs local physiotherapy practitioners who work with stroke patients to aid their recovery and help them to return to their communities. Abdullah and other practitioners I talked to strongly believed that one of the most beneficial activities they have carried out during the establishment of this project was an educational trip to learn from the experiences of fellow west Africans in Ghana, where rehabilitative professions had already been established. My initial discomfort with what seemed to be a desire for an exact copy of Western-centric practices to be implemented in his country, without making them contextually and culturally appropriate services, dissipated when I heard about the trip to Ghana. I was assured that local people in Sierra Leone, as in other Global South communities I work with such as Palestine, know that intercultural translation of practices from one context to another is best done when local knowledge and means of implementing that knowledge are incorporated and built on to enable occupation-based work to produce the best outcomes for their communities (Simaan, 2020).

People I talked to in Sierra Leone and other formerly and currently colonized nations have learnt historical lessons from colonization, slavery, and wars about the dangers of accepting outside "civilizational missions" that uncritically assume the superiority and universality of the Western models of health and community care provision. Based on historical and current experiences of education or aid provision by, for example, United Nations' institutions and international non-governmental organizations, it is clear that imposing the exact model of Western ways of life on Global South communities may be more harmful than helpful. Moreover, practitioners in Global South communities I visit tell me that they wish to offer community work and health services that suit their way of life, history, and context.

This important book is a seminal tool that I believe will help communities of praxis in the Global South to learn from each other, and to reflect on similarities and differences between their own situations and those they read about in these pages. Readers in the Global North can learn valuable lessons about everyday resistance, resilience, and representations of communities marginalized by forces such as capitalism, patriarchy, colonialism, racism and the climate crisis. The stories are told by leaders in occupational therapy from around the world, mainly from the Global South, and by some who work with Global South communities in the Global North.

Sheela Ivlev skilfully tells these stories by presenting in-depth conversations from interviews she conducted with practitioners involved with individuals and communities placed in unique circumstances. The interviewees' practices necessitated the application of high levels of creativity, critical reflexions, and resistance to the status quo to empower people to do the everyday activities they wished or needed to do in order for them to maintain their well-being and communities. The author lets the interviewees speak for themselves while offering illuminating observations and insights to help readers understand the context well.

This is an unashamedly political book that ushers in a decolonial era in the development of the disciplines of occupational therapy and occupational science. It joins earlier work which came out of South America and South Africa and which foregrounded non-anglophone and Global South epistemologies, as well as critiqued the assumed benefits in universally applying Eurocentric values and practices in communities that are marginalized by socioeconomic circumstances (e.g. Guajardo Córdoba, 2020; Lopes & Malfitano, 2021; Ramugondo, 2015). Developments in the last two decades in the discourses of occupational therapy and occupational science, such as the discussion of what has been termed "occupational justice" (Wilcock & Townsend, 2000), the publications of the *Occupational Therapies Without Borders* books (Kronenberg *et al.*, 2005), and the *Journal of Occupational Science's* Anti-Racism Pledge and Land Acknowledgement policy (Stanley *et al.*, 2020), have begun to advocate for community-focused work, equality, diversity, and inclusion in knowledge and practices. Although some voices and experiences from around the globe were highlighted in the above-mentioned publications, these discussions mainly came from scholars and authors from the Global North. What makes Sheela's book special is its origin and approach. The DisruptOT movement that Sheela founded and has led since 2021 has provided a needed safe space for Global South scholars and communities to raise important questions about the history of occupational therapy, its knowledge base, and its practices, from antiracist and anticolonial perspectives. These constructive conversations have paved the way for this book.

The author adopts a decolonial approach, which lets communities speak for themselves and provides a space for questioning and disrupting occupational therapy's core knowledge and practices. Concepts and practices that are core to occupational therapy and occupational science's knowledge in the Global North are questioned, such as "independence," "occupation," and even the title "occupational therapy." Take, for example, what Moussa says in Chapter 2 about the problematic use of the term "occupational therapy" in Palestine, where land and people are "occupied" and stripped off their rights and livelihood.

Other concepts are highlighted, such as "resistance," "representation," and "interdependence," which are offered as alternatives to mainstream practices by the interviewees, who are doing wonderful and necessary work in the most difficult of circumstances. In Chapter 5, Ann in Ghana tells us how "dicey" the use of "independence" as a goal for occupational therapy intervention is in a communal society such as Ghana. She instead speaks of the importance of "communal love," sacrifice, and reciprocating. Documenting the stories in this book is a step in the right direction toward learning and reflecting on more equitable and inclusive knowledge and practice. In the words of Boavuntura de Sosa Santos, this book represents "an invitation to a much larger experience of the world as one's own and thus to a much broader company in the task of transforming the world into a more equal and more diverse world" (2014, p.240).

This book will certainly be included in my curriculum, and should be on the reading list of all learners, educators, and scholars of occupational therapy, occupational science, and other health and social care disciplines and community workers concerned with decolonizing the Western-centric knowledge base and with making their societies more equitable and healthy. I congratulate Sheela, the DisruptOT community, and, in particular, the interviewees, who are leading the way in dreaming about and remaking the worlds of occupational therapy and occupational science, and their own local communities, a safer space for daily living and flourishing, despite all the oppressive historical, global, and local contextual factors that heavily restrict their lives. I look forward to continuing these constructive conversations with colleagues around the world to make occupational therapy and occupational science, and our shared world, kinder and more inclusive for everyone. This book and the DisruptOT movement help us to hope for, and dream about, a world in which we might not even need an institution with a history in which one dominant view of the world takes precedence and therefore leads to exclusive access and gatekept knowledge creation. Just like the Black Lives Matter movement's calls for abolishing the police, or the global refugee solidarity movement's call to abolish borders, we perhaps need to begin a discussion about abolishing occupational therapy. Instead, we may wish to frame our justice- and occupation-focused work as activism that invites everybody to take part, rather than maintaining a small circle of elite practitioners, qualified by elite universities and regulated by elite bodies, all of which were part of a historical pattern of exclusive Eurocentric knowledge production and practices. By not carrying the historical associations of exclusivity, the praxis of occupation and justice-based activism will welcome partners and collaborators who might otherwise not join this project of making the world a more safe and accessible space, in which individuals and societies are free to take part in meaningful and purposeful daily lives as they wish or need to.

Juman Simaan (he/his/him) is a Palestinian living in the UK. He is an associate professor of occupational therapy at Edinburgh Napier University. Juman's scholarship focuses on Global South means of knowing and doing, and on decolonial and transformational approaches to education. Juman is an associate editor for the Journal of Occupational Science, *and has worked together with board members of the journal to agree on an antiracist pledge and land acknowledgement policy as small steps in the ongoing collective effort towards the decolonization of the discipline of occupational science.*

References

American Occupational Therapy Association. (2020). *2019 Workforce and Salary Survey*. https://library.aota.org/AOTA-Workforce-Salary-Survey-2019.

Black, R.M. (2002). "Occupational therapy's dance with diversity." *American Journal of Occupational Therapy*, 56(2): 140–148. doi:10.5014/ajot.56.2.140.

Césaire, A. (1984). *Notebook of a Return to the Native Land*. Berkeley, CA: University of California Press.

Grenier, M.L. (2020). "Cultural competency and the reproduction of White supremacy in occupational therapy education." *Health Education Journal*, 79(6): 633–644. doi:10.1177/0017896920902515.

Guajardo Córdoba, A. (2020). "About new forms of colonization in occupational therapy: Reflections on the idea of occupational justice from a critical-political philosophy perspective. *Cadernos Brasileiros de Terapia Ocupacional*, 28(4). https://doi.org/10.4322/2526-8910.ctoARF2175.

Kronenberg, F., Simó Algado, S., & Pollard, N. (eds) (2005). *Occupational Therapy Without Borders: Learning from the Spirit of Survivors*. Edinburgh: Elsevier.

Lopes, E.R. & Malfitano, P.A. (2021). *Social Occupational Therapy: Theoretical and Practical Designs*. Edinburgh: Elsevier.

Ramugondo, E.L. (2015). "Occupational consciousness." *Journal of Occupational Science*, 22(4): 488–501. https://doi.org/10.1080/14427591.2015.1042516.

Santos, B.S. (2014). *Epistemologies of the South: Justice Against Epistemicide*. Oxford: Routledge.

Simaan, J. (2020). "Decolonising occupational science education through learning activities based on a study from the Global South." *Journal of Occupational Science*, 27(3): 432–442. doi: 10.1080/14427591.2020.1780937.

Stanley, M., Rogers, S., Forwell, S., Hocking, C. *et al.* (2020). "A pledge to mobilize against racism." *Journal of Occupational Science*, 27(3): 295–295. https://dopi.org/10.1080/14427591.2020.1793446.

Wilcock, A.A. & Townsend, E. (2000). "Occupational justice: Occupational terminology interactive dialogue." *Journal of Occupational Science*, 7(2): 84–86.

Acknowledgements

I am forever grateful to old friends and new who trusted me to tell their stories, connected me with their peers, offered support and encouragement, and without whom, there would be no book and no DisruptOT.

Thank you to Shawn Borsky for providing guidance and inspiration throughout the cover design process.

To my husband, Alex, thank you for your brutal honesty and endless hours of unpaid editing. I hope you learned what occupational therapy is.

With my parents showing me the meaning of community, connection, and care, I could cultivate all of these relationships. They taught me to live as if the world has no borders, speak out about injustices, and not wait to take action. I owe them everything.

INTRODUCTION

Despite a globally connected world, occupational therapy remains disconnected. There aren't enough opportunities to learn about the profession worldwide in school or practice. With over 100 countries offering occupational therapy services, we are mostly exposed to the same handful of Western approaches.

This book grew out of a movement I started in 2021 called DisruptOT (www.disruptot.org). After a decade of not feeling as if I belonged in the profession and recognizing that much of what I was taught to do made no sense in my own life, I sought to connect virtually with global peers during an uncontrolled pandemic.

Our conversations and debates turned into bonds, and the possibilities of what to do with the knowledges we gained of our everyday doings flourished. So, in 2021, with the help of volunteers worldwide, we organized the inaugural DisruptOT Community Summit, with the theme of building community. On August 7 and 8, we held a two-day free live forum with speakers representing 21 countries. The online event covered healing, antiracism, decolonization, gender, sexuality, mental health, and building community, with hundreds of people joining us from different parts of the world. Since then, we have been offering free monthly educational and networking opportunities with international speakers and attendees from various health backgrounds, many with lived experience in the areas they discuss. Our priority is to highlight global voices, make access to this critical knowledge free and accessible to all, and compensate labor. We pay our speakers fairly and generously because we value them and the gifts they offer us. With help from hundreds of individuals and several organizations, we use a mutual aid model to collect funds that go directly to speakers.

In this book, we are going to step outside what we know and travel to several countries to learn stories that haven't been shared before.

I wrote this book to document new histories in occupational therapy and share narratives of global resistance and representation. We will learn different ways of being and doing. And we will be asked to reflect critically on what we think we know and take actions to grow beyond that.

This book does not offer easy solutions, nor will it make us cultural experts. On the contrary, we will discover individual accounts that give us a small window into occupational therapy in each country we visit. These stories are meant to pique our interest and encourage us to learn and do more.

The people featured in this book trusted me to share their stories, as have the many speakers at our global events. This work is needed, and DisruptOT participants have told us that we offer them opportunities to:

- build communities and connections with people worldwide
- move beyond the Eurocentric knowledge base
- gain globally informed perspectives
- challenge assumptions, beliefs, and prior learnings
- feel hope that the profession can be and do better.

Each chapter tells a unique story, introduces occupational therapy in various contexts, and shares personalities, joy, and pain. Read each chapter, complete the reflection and action prompts, and get motivated to connect and build a community to disrupt with.

CHAPTER 1

UGANDA: Victor Alochi

Victor Alochi is a man with one name. Alochi means victor. He is from the northern part of Uganda, west of the Nile River.

I first noticed his work on Twitter, a picture of an adapted toilet seat built from a plastic chair with the seat cut out to go over a pit latrine. For a type of toilet that requires one to squat down to use, his adapted seat would make it easier for the person to use the toilet with less assistance and more privacy. Scrolling through his account, @OTVictorAlochi, you see the many devices he has innovated to help people in rural Ugandan communities more easily participate in their daily occupations. He has built corner seats and

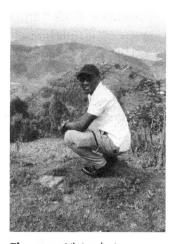

Figure 1.1: Victor between Mount Muhavura, Mount Mgahinga, and Mount Sabyinyo, the point where Uganda, Congo, and Rwanda meet

orthoses out of cardboard and newspaper, parallel bars, accessible animal pens, and showers from nearby trees, and many more critical inventions with easy-to-find local materials.

As he works long days without breaks, it is a challenge to connect with Victor. When I attempt to arrange the interview, he has just worked two weeks straight without a break because of the escalating crisis in Congo, resulting in a recent surge of refugees entering

Uganda. Victor has been where he is most needed, supporting people with disabilities coming into the country with barely any belongings and no necessary medical equipment to participate in daily life.

The crisis continues, but he manages to get a day off so we can meet virtually. Victor begins with a much-needed geography and history lesson. He tells the story of the two sons of King Olum, Gipir and Labongo. There was a disagreement between the two brothers, and Labongo and his family went to the area east of the Nile, moving southwards and then eastwards into Kenya. Gipir and Labongo are the ancestral fathers of all Luo, which is why the dialects and languages of various tribes remain relatively similar.

Uganda is divided into four regions and almost 140 districts. "Victor Victor," he calls himself, laughing, is Ugandan by nationality, Alur by tribe. From within the tribe of Alur, he is a Jonam, "the people of the lake or river." These valuable introductory teachings tell me about Victor, where he is from, and later will explain how he can communicate with people from surrounding countries.

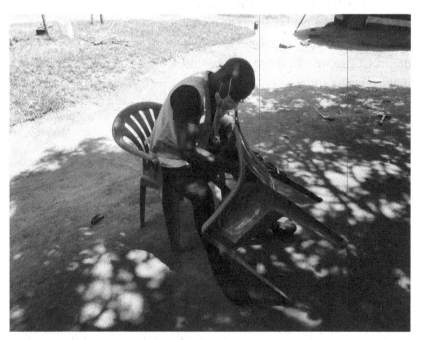

Figure 1.2: Victor carving out the seat of a plastic chair to build an adapted toilet seat

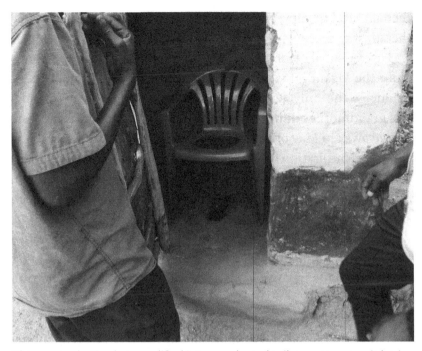

Figure 1.3: Plastic chair modified into an adapted toilet seat over a pit latrine

Born in the north of Uganda and raised in the center of the country, he grew up with his grandmother, whom he calls mom, as his mother left when he was six months old. Raised in a rural area with no hospital services, he moved to the capital city of Kampala in 1998 to receive treatment after a dog bit him.

As a five-year-old child, he went with his grandmother for a burial service at her ancestral home. There weren't many cars back then, so they walked 40 kilometers and slept by the roadside. As they walked, she was suffering from knee, back, and hip pain. Those cries are forever etched in his memory. When they returned home, her pain continued throughout her life.

After high school, Victor considered medicine and surgery, not knowing about occupational therapy. He didn't receive a government scholarship for university and couldn't afford to pay privately. So, he went to his teachers and asked for other options. They recommended getting a diploma instead of a bachelor's degree to qualify for a government scholarship. For his application, he listed pharmacy first, then physical therapy, and occupational therapy last. Occupational therapy was selected for him.

He graduated in July 2016 with an occupational therapy diploma from the Uganda Institute of Allied Health and Management Sciences, the only occupational therapy program in Uganda. His grandmother didn't have a chance to see him graduate. She passed away in May of the same year. In his graduation speech, he shared his inspiration for finishing the program—his grandmother. Though he regrets not being able to help her, he sees the value in his education and training because of all the people he has been able to help since.

The first brief clinical placement was in his first year at St. Francis Hospital, Buluba in Mayuge District, which was built to treat leprosy patients in eastern Uganda. During his second year, the Occupational Therapy Africa Regional Group (OTARG) held a conference in Uganda in 2015. It was the first conference he attended as well as presented at. He spoke about the role of occupational therapy with leprosy patients, including home modifications. He recalls working with a woman with leprosy who left her home in Sudan to go to Uganda for treatment and didn't want to go back home because she couldn't shower at home and didn't want her grandchildren to bathe her. It was then Victor created the tipi tap shower, a standing shower frame distributing water from a jerrycan above, and she was able to return home. There is no running water in these areas. Water is pumped from a well or collected in nearby streams and ponds.

He is still trying to figure out how to bring the water up without a pump, which is too expensive. He shows me a large plastic water basin, most commonly used for bathing in rural areas. Squatting down, both hands are cupped to distribute water along the body while the basin sits on the floor. Modifications include using a cup for distributing water and a platform to hold the basin higher as part of his interventions.

Some of his other inventions include replacing a broken wheelchair seat with a plastic chair, building long-handled brooms, and setting up foot- and hand-activated hand-washing stations in regions with no running water.

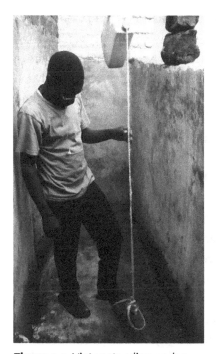 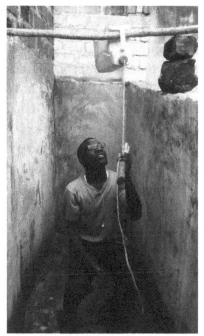

Figure 1.4: Victor standing under tipi tap shower using foot control to distribute water from jerrycan above. This set-up is typically used for someone with an upper limb injury or amputation

Figure 1.5: Victor sitting under tipi tap shower using hand control to distribute water from jerrycan above. This set-up is typically used for someone with a lower limb injury or amputation

He completed internships each semester all over the country in various settings. In his third and final year, he went to western Uganda to work in a rehabilitation hospital for children, including doing community-based work. He credits his problem solving skills and creative thinking to the knowledge he learned here with his mentor, Ambrose Gasanga.

The occupational therapy textbooks he studied were all Western, as most were donated by foreign, mostly British, visitors. In 2010, the seminal African context textbook, *Occupational Therapy: An African Perspective*, was published (Alers & Crouch, 2010). It was edited by Westerners with many African contributors. A copy was donated to the occupational therapy program in 2015 during the OTARG conference. Victor purchased his own copy in 2018 at the

World Federation of Occupational Therapists (WFOT) Congress in South Africa. More recently, textbooks have been written by African occupational therapists in South Africa, including *Concepts in Occupational Therapy: Understanding Southern Perspectives* (Galvaan & Ramugondo, 2017), another book Victor purchased at WFOT, and brought back to Uganda. *Disabled Village Children* (Werner, 1987) is one of the most helpful books he's used in community practice. When he was studying, there was one copy of the book with only a few pages remaining, as people had taken the helpful pages out to use. Now it's available freely online.

Specialty training or certification is not available in Uganda. They are generalists, but Victor considers himself a community occupational therapist based on his interests. There is a greater need for occupational therapy in the community, and that's where he chooses to be.

After graduating, he volunteered for two months and got a job at an addiction center. Part of their community work was to familiarize locals with their programs. Every Sunday, they went to churches to teach people about addiction. He was there for three years until opening Ebenezer Rehabilitation Clinic after recognizing he could address needs in the community. This catered to the elderly, as that had been his drive for entering this profession. He went to people's homes in the village without any cost to them. He charged for clinic-based services to pay overhead expenses, allowing for pro bono community-based services. When the pandemic hit, people were afraid to come to the clinic, and they didn't get any clients for three months. Then, their rent was raised, so he had to leave the facility and close the clinic.

He currently works for Humanity & Inclusion, an international nonprofit, non-governmental organization. Initially, his work was with ultra-poor people in northern Uganda in the refugee settlement, specifically helping individuals with disabilities graduate from school. He was also doing in-home and workplace modifications. One modification was for an older woman who raised goats for a living and could no longer put her goats in the pen because of her disability. He adapted the hut structure, and the woman could enter and exit without pain. This was supposed to be a three-year project, but with fewer donations during the pandemic, the program was cut after a year and a half.

He then moved to a refugee holding center because of the instability in the Democratic Republic of Congo. There has been an influx of close to 42,000 refugees entering Uganda. Refugees come across the border to a holding center and then move to a transit center when they decide to stay and move to a settlement. It is their choice, and they can remain in the holding center until they decide to either return home or settle in this new country.

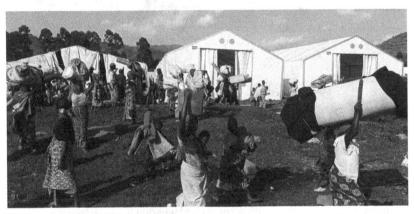

Figure 1.6: People moving about the holding center

Victor's job is to support refugees with disabilities coming to Uganda to participate fully in all aspects of life. So, he advocates for accessibility. When he first went to the holding facility, he met a person who hadn't been able to bathe in a week because there was nowhere to sit and shower for someone with lower limb amputations.

He is the only occupational therapist in the holding facility and completes accessibility audits, including focus groups of residents with disabilities, to find out what is not accessible. He advises on accessibility modifications to current structures and makes recommendations for new ones being built. Because of the lack of resources and a temporary living environment, the modifications he makes are simple and show people that once they move to a settlement or return home, they can still have access to similar equipment.

Everyone benefits from universal design. I encourage Victor to study engineering if he ever returns to school because he is a creative innovator and problem solver who builds things people need with limited resources available. He excitedly laughs and smiles, leaning into the camera. The possibility is intriguing.

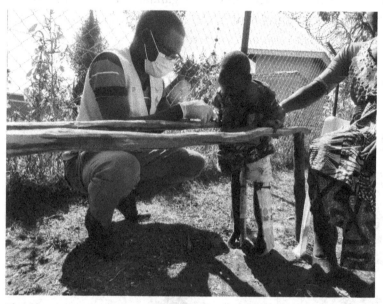

Figure 1.7: Victor working with a small child wearing lower extremity orthoses he made from cardboard and newspapers using the parallel bars he built from nearby trees to work on the child's mobility

People often return home from the settlements, but because of the war, many eventually return to the settlement. He has to bear this in mind when educating and training them, including the uncertainty of their future. The needs of the people in the holding center are often immediate and can't wait until they are settled, like the inaccessible toileting and bathing facilities.

The facility is 6 kilometers from Rwanda and 9 kilometers from Congo. When the refugee crisis began, he was working until 9pm every night. The day can begin at various times: 7am for awareness sessions to find people who need support before they move and make them aware of services available to them. On settlement relocation days, they have to start at 6am. On population count days, they start at 4am. He sleeps in a rented guest house nearby, shared with other workers. Travel home, about 800 kilometers, would take a full day, so he stays at the guest house for months, with little time off. The last time he went home, his one-year-old daughter didn't recognize him and ran away as he tried to approach her. His work is his life right now.

Refugees live in enormous tents at the holding center. Each tent has a shelter leader and houses up to 150 people. They act as ambassadors for the needs of people within their tents. These shelter leaders make referrals for therapy services. There is also a physical therapist on site, and together they train community-based facilitators who act as interpreters to identify people who might benefit from services. When he does follow-ups, he goes to these 77 shelters one by one.

Here he tries to invent equipment they cannot access, creating efficient processes to get everyone who needs support seen. He also trains people who come from other organizations. There are about 17,000 people in the holding center, with one occupational therapist, Victor. Last Monday, 50 people were waiting to work with him. Everyone was educated on the services available, and to prioritize care, he asked people who had been seen before to return another day.

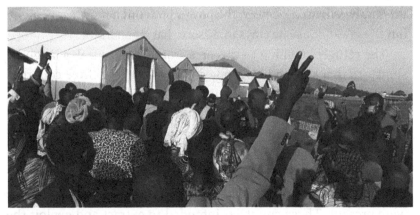

Figure 1.8: Holding center residents being oriented to services available to them

When Victor explains occupational therapy, he insists on using the term, even though the residents and even medics don't know what it is or what he does. He explains that he works with people with mental and physical challenges using activities as treatment. His role is to design or look at things around them to see how they can be done better, more independently, or without pain. It's more difficult for people in rural communities to understand what occupational therapy is because of their lack of exposure to these services, so he helps them see that he works with people using the activities that they do every day.

When working in local communities in Kiryandongo, he spoke many languages, including Luo, Kiswahili, Luganda, Nubi, and English. Many languages are spoken throughout the country, but knowing Swahili makes it easier to communicate with many people. For example, in one hospital, he would speak Alur, Acholi and Langi (Luo). He wasn't fluent, but because of shared ancestry and root language, he was able to pick up on everyday words and communicate easily. He is often the interpreter for his colleagues because he speaks so many languages.

The power suddenly goes out, and it is pitch black on the screen except for the reflection on Victor's glasses from his phone screen. Victor asks if I get outages too. I tell him I don't but spending time throughout my life in India, I was used to having the power go out randomly. Where he is now, the power goes out almost every night, but the guest house he stays in, Kisoro, has a generator.

The refugees coming to this area from Congo speak a language similar to that spoken in Uganda and Rwanda. The three countries used to be the same, but the Partition of Africa, also called the Scramble for Africa, separated them into distinct countries, as is the case with most of Africa's borders. Following the Berlin conference of 1884–85, European countries invaded, colonized, and divided land in Africa, though much of coastal Africa was already colonized. Major European countries were invited to the conference, but no Africans were present. These countries intended to extract and exploit the precious resources that made Africa so valuable, and to civilize Africans via Christianity. Locals were forced to pay taxes to the colonial governments that took over their land, and were often killed or had their extremities chopped off if they couldn't make the payments (Gjersø, 2015).

When we look at maps, we see borders, but they don't naturally occur. Shared language cannot be divided by a manufactured border. In Uganda, the common language is Kifumbira; in Congo, it is Kinyabwisha; in Rwanda, it is Kinyarwanda; in Burundi, it is Kirundi. Their accents might differ, but the same language, shared cultures, and brutal histories connect the people.

Going deeper into the neighboring countries, languages change. Victor is trying to learn the basics of this shared language to communicate with people in the holding center. He now knows some general phrases. Community-based interpreters from the local area in Uganda interpret the languages of residents and workers.

The power comes back on, and I can see Victor again, wearing a maroon t-shirt and glasses with a buzzed haircut and faint mustache visible. He's sitting by the front door of the guest house, which opens a couple of times as his housemates enter. Behind him is a long green curtain with block patterns of a giraffe family. A comfortable contrast to the images he shares of the holding center.

He brings his work tablet up to the camera and shows me pictures. In one, outside, surrounded by large white tents, a big group of people is waiting to be seen, sitting on rows of long benches or standing. They are facing the center, surrounding two people standing, one in a bright yellow vest, the community facilitator, who is translating for Victor, standing next to him wearing a mask. Flipping through photos, I see rows of people attentively listening and a bench off to the side with a row of people holding brand-new canes. These were imported and provided to residents. He makes the things they cannot access.

I reflect on the immense privilege I experienced working at the local Veterans Affairs hospital in San Francisco, where I could walk into a closet and hand walkers, canes, wheelchairs, commodes, and smaller assistive devices to veterans when needed. Anything more expensive or complex required completing a form, and they would soon receive what they needed free of charge to their home.

It's now 10pm, it's been two hours, and Victor has to work in the morning. I have more to ask and don't want to keep him from resting. Victor enjoys the conversation and sharing his work and is happy to continue so we talk for almost another hour.

Some people walk over, and others are picked up by trucks to cross the border. Those who decide to return to Congo have to walk. As we are speaking, the border is under the control of rebels that defeated government control across the border. They have stopped the entry of cars into Congo but allow the entry and exit of asylum seekers. It's not safe for people to go back because of the attacks. There is no guess as to when the conflict will end.

Uganda is known as the Pearl of Africa, and he describes it as the most beautiful country in the world. It's full of nature, hills and plains and has the most lakes in Africa. He points in various directions around him and tells me where there are local lakes, including one on the top of Mount Muhavura, which means direction. From the top of the mountain, you can see Uganda, Congo, and Rwanda. Many people come to Uganda to see mountain gorillas. There are just over 1000 remaining in the world. He shares images from his phone sent by his supervisor today, who was on the road from West Nile. I see elephants, buffalo, boar, waterbucks, and lush green vegetation.

Despite other countries being more specialized and advanced, Uganda has prioritized culture and context in occupational therapy practice. Modifications and interventions are culturally accepted, culturally adapted, and locally available. They work with things in the community that are familiar to users. When Victor modifies and adapts equipment, he shows the community, so they learn how to do it. He aims to make it sustainable, so if an occupational therapist isn't available, they can do it themselves.

I hope there are more opportunities for people to learn about Victor's work, as many practitioners need to understand the limitations in remote communities. Some international organizations donate equipment like wheelchairs that are not meant for the terrain, and there is no material to maintain them. We should be helping communities work together when therapists are limited and helping them support each other instead of trying to intervene with what we think they need.

Victor hopes occupational therapy in Uganda can catch up to the level in Western countries, with PhD programs, advanced-level practice, and more evidenced-based practice and research being published outside the country. He wants the global occupational therapy community to be more connected and to collaborate with countries struggling to set up programs. An exchange program could facilitate global learning, sharing of ideas, and cultural exchange. After the OTARG conference, he started a WhatsApp group to organize student leaders in Africa, which later became a space for practitioners across Africa to share best practices and work through complex cases.

His advice to readers is to be proud of being an occupational therapist and work *with* people, not *on* them. He gives an example of a woman using a commode bucket to carry beans from the market because while the therapist had decided this was what the family member needed, it was actually not helping them with the problem. We should be on the same level, exchanging ideas, working in harmony, appreciating each other, and ensuring we don't create a dependence on therapists.

Now that you have read Victor's story, please take some time to think about occupational therapy in your context. You are invited to write down your thoughts and ideas.

SUGGESTED NEXT STEPS

Reflection: What do you consider to be community-based care? How can occupational therapy in your region better reach people where they are?

Action: What innovation might support community practice in your region? Without worrying about barriers, identify something that should exist to fill the gaps in community care. This is your chance to invent something.

References

Alers, V. & Crouch, R. (eds) (2010). *Occupational Therapy: An African Perspective.* Johannesburg: Sarah Shorten Publishers.

Galvaan, R. & Ramugondo, E.L. (2017). *Concepts in Occupational Therapy: Understanding Southern Perspectives.* Manipal: Manipal University Press.

Gjersø, J. (2015). "The Scramble for East Africa: British motives reconsidered, 1884–95." *The Journal of Imperial and Commonwealth History*, 43(5): 831–860, doi: 10.1080/03086534.2015.1026131.

Werner, D. (1987). *Disabled Village Children.* Palo Alto, CA: The Hesperian Foundation.

CHAPTER 2

PALESTINE: Moussa Abu Mostafa

Moussa Abu Mostafa is a 55-year-old Palestinian man. He is mostly bald, with a serious face that rarely breaks into a smile, a freshly graying beard, and a dark mustache. It's late Sunday evening in Gaza, and he is wearing a starched powder blue button-up shirt after a day of work.

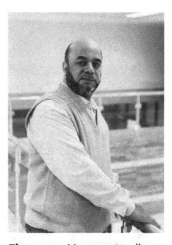

Friday and Saturday are the usual days off in Palestine, a majority Muslim country. Friday is a day for communal worship, where people go to the mosque to pray and take in *khutbah*, weekly teachings on community concerns led by the imam. This person leads prayer and is often the head of the community. Moussa practices his faith,

Figure 2.1: Moussa standing over a glass and metal railing

values community, and learns about Islamic teachings emphasizing respect and how to contribute to society during the weekly *khutbah*.

Moussa is a father of six children, a husband, an occupational therapist, a researcher, and a lecturer. Raising his eyebrows and sitting up taller, he adds, "I was born here in Palestine, not outside Palestine. That is very important." I later recognize the significance of this declaration. Although Moussa lives in the Gaza Strip in Palestine, he has had opportunities to leave and live a safe and easier life. Still, he chooses to stay because remaining at home is how he believes he will make the most impact on the lives of his people.

I ask him to tell me about his home. "In Gaza, cultures differ and integrate with nature. Wherever you look, you find what attracts you to talk about; it's modern and old. It is a civilization that gathers everything beautifully. The sound of mosques and church bells overwhelms you, and the laughs of children, elders' conversation, and their pearls of wisdom amaze you. Look at Gaza's harbor at night; it is a piece of the lighting moon. It is Gaza despite the difference and damage."

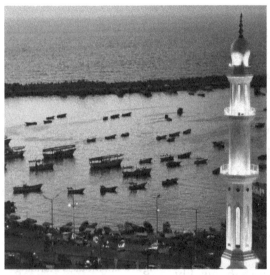

Figure 2.2: Harbor of Gaza at twilight

Palestine is divided into two territories—Gaza and the West Bank— with two governments and two distinct systems. During our conversation, he never gets into the politics between Israel and Palestine, never places any blame. Instead, he talks about Nelson Mandela choosing forgiveness in the face of apartheid and imprisonment, and looking towards South Africa's future, and he emphasizes, in his words, that "punishment, violence, revenge, will only further the divide."

Moussa wants unity for every generation and believes that if people can move past their individual experiences, forgive those who harmed them, and prioritize peace for their community, they have a chance to move forward and find peace. In addition, the struggle for independence requires a health system that supports the struggle. This means that even occupational therapy needs to put community first by prioritizing health for all people. Currently, Palestinians injured by Israelis have their treatment paid for. Palestinians injured by Palestinians are required to pay for themselves.

There is much more to learn outside this text and our conversation. In 1917, with the Balfour Declaration, Britain declared its support to make Palestine a home for Jewish people despite it already being home to mostly Arabs, bolstering Zionism. Nazi persecution of Jews in Eastern Europe resulted in major migration to Palestine. Palestine was the only former Ottoman territory not to gain full independence, and the massive immigration resulted in long-standing violence. Over the years, Israel became an independent state, a distinction that Palestine still does not hold globally. Israel has taken over most Palestinian territory, occupying the separated West Bank and Gaza Strip, pushing out much of the Arab population, or trapping them in one of these open-air prisons if they remain (United Nations, n.d.). Ethnic cleansing and displacement of Palestinians has further shifted the demographics (Pappe, 2006). Occupational apartheid may be the best way to describe occupation in a country physically divided, with people displaced and unable to go home or access basic necessities. On one side, there is freedom, safety, access to essential resources, and more. Directly across, in what used to be historical Palestine, and now is occupied territories, life is different.

Israel controls access in and out of Gaza, by land, sea, and air. It decides who can leave and who cannot. The majority of Palestinian people cannot leave. Control extends to restricting necessities needed to survive, resulting in high unemployment and limited access to food, clean water, electricity, materials to reconstruct destroyed buildings and infrastructure, schools, medical care, financial services, and places of religious significance. This has resulted in poverty for about 56 percent of Palestinians in Gaza and turned over 60 percent into refugees. They cannot leave this open-air prison to return home (Al Jazeera, 2022; Humaid, 2022).

Despite the violent realities of everyday life, Moussa's story is one of resistance. He studied electrical engineering for three years at Birzeit University until all universities abruptly closed due to the Intifada, a collective uprising against the Israeli occupation of Palestine beginning in 1987 and ending in 1993. Israeli forces closed all educational institutions, yet people resisted and came together to have classes in gardens. The Intifada seriously impacted the lives of Palestinians, resulting in massive injuries and civilian casualties (United Nations, n.d.; Naser-Najjab, 2020). Moussa's most meaningful occupations were seized: his studies and hope for a future. Life was brought to a halt by the Intifada. After two years of university closures, Moussa realized that the school would not reopen. He moved to Greece, a country welcoming Palestinians. After spending a year learning Greek, he went to the Embassy in Athens to register for university. There he discussed the needs of the Gaza Strip. With limited options and hope for a fresh start, he was advised to take occupational therapy, which he did not know anything about at the time, but agreed to move forward as it was something he could bring home to benefit his people.

His eyes glowing with pride, Moussa recounts being the only foreigner in his program and graduating at the top of the class. The mood shifts back and forth as he shares his success while mourning the years lost. Moussa had solid opportunities for a life and career in Greece, but after completing his studies, he was ready to return to life in Palestine, exclaiming, "I didn't wait one minute." Though he felt supported in Greece, he was prepared to return to his roots immediately. He returned home as the first person in the Gaza Strip with a bachelor's degree in occupational therapy. Failure was common for Palestinian students studying abroad. With relief and satisfaction, Moussa shares that he felt rewarded and made up for the lost time when returning home by securing the job he wanted.

El Wafa Medical Rehabilitation Hospital is the first medical rehabilitation hospital in Gaza, and Moussa worked there for 25 years from 1996. In his first role as an occupational therapist, he covered inpatient and outpatient neuro rehabilitation. Currently, he is the head of occupational therapy at the Hamad Medical Rehabilitation Hospital, which is funded by Qatar Foundation for Development. It has inpatient, day treatment, outpatient, neuro rehabilitation, orthopedics, and additional services not available at El Wafa, like prosthetics and hearing aids. Additionally, he is a part-time lecturer and has been for most of his career. Moussa has also worked in community rehabilitation and provided community-based education.

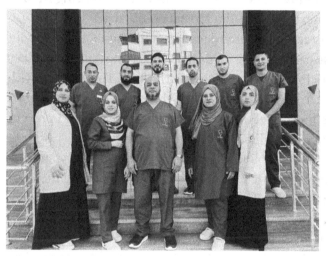

Figure 2.3: The occupational therapy department at Hamad Medical Rehabilitation Hospital

Moussa's love for education pushed him to complete a master's degree. He had to rule out programs in the United States as they would not allow him to do research from his home country, and he would have had to move. Finding an affordable program at Stellenbosch University in South Africa, he completed his research back home. With a strong sense of duty to help his people, to raise their voices, he knows no one will come from the outside to help them. He was born in Palestine and reiterates, "I am from the context" and, "I am one of them."

Health education and participation of people in Gaza with spinal cord injuries (SCI) are his research priorities. He recognized a gap in research and resources to reduce complications and include families in treatment. When examining discharges from rehabilitation hospitals in Gaza, Moussa noticed that patients lacked resources, were unable to complete inpatient rehabilitation, had difficulty with daily life, were prone to complications like pressure injuries, had poor inclusion in the community, and subsequently returned to the hospital for preventable causes. He also noticed that girls in Islamic communities with SCI did not receive an adequate education compared to boys with SCI. Notable occupations affected include participating in prayer and related rituals critical to being Arab in the Islamic context of Gaza (Abu Mostafa *et al.*, 2023).

Participatory action research demands "nothing about us without us." The people participating in his research are not subjects; "They are active participants. I'm studying with them, I'm learning with them, we are learning with each other," he insists. When resources are scarce, the most effective way to promote health and prevent illness and injury is the dissemination of information.

Moussa researches for liberation, "when publishing and your work reaches outside, you are free. [You] influence people around the globe without restrictions... Like the restrictions that killed my schoolmates." Noticing my pain and discomfort, he remarks, "I can see this in your face, but this is reality." Research is freedom, and research that uncovers inequities and occupational injustices improves the lives of the next generation. He explains, "Writing this work is important because when people are reading it around the world, you are free. You are free from the colonized Gaza Strip. From all the restrictions. The pain of the past and present. Wherever the paper is read, our roots will extend to our country of origin."

Collaboration, lived experience, and research benefit his people. This is why he funds his own research, practices as an occupational therapist, leads his occupational therapy team, and teaches. Research documents the struggle and records the barriers, inequities, and injustices faced by Palestinians. Documented evidence means people will notice, offering hope that something will change. Moussa's research, teaching, practice, and life illuminate grave inequities and generational occupational injustices.

Research is not apolitical. For example, spinal cord injuries are blamed on attacks by Palestinians, though there is no evidence for this. In addition, Palestinian culture and religion differ from Western and Christian religions as Palestinians are primarily Muslim, and their average age is much younger. The median age for the Gaza Strip is 19, an all-time high for the country, whereas the world average is almost a decade higher (CEIC, n.d.). Studying the gaps and searching for appropriate practice models that fit the Palestinian culture and context, Moussa developed and tested the *Spinal Cord Injury Activities of Daily Living Education Manual*, an educational tool co-produced with people with SCI in Gaza.

When looking for a PhD program, Moussa had to consider traveling outside the Gaza Strip, which is risky and near impossible for most. He speaks of being humiliated with mistreatment and unnecessary delays when trying to leave or return, and being at the mercy of guards. The journey is unsafe, and he could be killed, beaten, or taken to prison in a surrounding country. With the Gaza airport destroyed and access points closed, options to leave or enter are limited and dangerous. Moussa refers to his homeland as a "big prison." Yet, he brings up the war in Ukraine and his concern for lives lost and forever affected. Having life changed forever and choices taken away are things he deeply understands.

"They destroyed the whole country. It's not a street. It's not one building. It's not a room. It's a whole country with a history, with a people, with a nation, with children, with everything. They need hundreds of years to fix this, and they never will because many people were killed. Innocent people were killed. They will not come back to life."

We pause to reflect on the significance of these words and his experiences. It's been two hours, the time I initially requested for this interview, and many questions remain. I ask if we can continue despite it being nine in the evening, and knowing he had been working today and would need to return in the morning. Moussa requests five minutes to pray, leaves the room, and promptly returns.

Arabic, English, Hebrew, and Greek are the languages he speaks and practices in. وظيفي (*wadifi*) is the Arabic word used to describe occupation, meaning work or filling your time with something.

A common phrase used in various Arab countries to explain occupational therapy is treating by work, a backward translation from العلاج المهني (āl ʿilāji almehniu). The Arabic-speaking world uses different words to describe occupation depending on where they are explaining it.

Moussa finds inadequate all words used to explain occupation and occupational therapy in the languages he is familiar with. He compares the phrases "colonization" and "decolonization" with the controversy around the term "occupational therapy," clarifying that colonization isn't inherently bad; it is simply investing in empty land without people. However, that meaning changes when the people of these lands become marginalized, displaced, neglected, and stripped of their rights and choices, when they are "removed from the map, and their existence is no longer." This is critical to occupational therapy. Decolonization is the opposite, assuring the rights of the people, participation, building partnerships, and supporting their existence. He speaks of the colonization of Palestine, of having decisions, choices, and freedom taken away. People were given work but not opportunities when their land was taken over. He is still talking about occupation, just not how I'm used to understanding it in practice. He tells me the colonizers of the land "taught us how to plant trees, but they...kept the good seeds." Seeds are significant, as agriculture is how Palestinians have sustained themselves. With land taken, roads blocked, and water scarce, farmers are separated from their crops, crops are threatened, and so are the livelihoods of Palestinians. As is echoed in Moussa's research, for people to succeed, they must be part of the work, and the power must be shared.

Three hours into our almost four-hour interview, Moussa's screen freezes. Moments after, he drops off the video call. Several minutes later, his face appears on the screen with a formal living room behind him decorated with fringed curtains and dried flowers in a vase. The power went out, he explains. Moussa is stoic, rarely breaking his serious expression. I have a feeling he was relieved that I stayed on the call waiting for his return as he jumped right into explaining the electricity situation. I'm relieved that he returned. We have a lot more to discuss.

The electrical grid in the Gaza Strip runs eight hours on and eight hours off, going up to 12 hours without power in the summer. There are additional power cuts due to frequent bombardment of civilian infrastructure. Some households use generators to keep the electricity running, but using them is not without risk or cost at almost eight times the standard rate, making access difficult and extremely cost prohibitive for the average household. As Moussa recounts various injuries and deaths related to generator accidents in his country, his brows furrow, his forehead wrinkles, and his head bows as he mourns the lives lost. The heaviness dissipates as he shares that technology has since improved, and he has access to safer generators. Resources like electricity, food, fuel, clean water, and other essentials are limited in Palestine.

Outages are a reality of life, making engagement in daily occupations unnecessarily precarious. The nightly routines of cooking, doing chores, reading, and studying occur in the dark. Electricity means the ability to study thoroughly, and education means a higher likelihood of a better life. Moussa prioritizes his children's education above all else, which has required sacrifice over many years.

There are many barriers to providing the best care. The most significant obstructions are political and economic. Though Gaza has had occupational therapy licensure since 1997, before the West Bank and much of the Arab world, and it is a respected independent health profession, there is still no bachelor's degree, only a diploma program. There are challenges to improving occupational therapy education and training as people cannot leave, and outsiders cannot come in to share best practices. Many have taken significant risks in going back and forth between Gaza and the West Bank, where there are bachelor's and master's programs in occupational therapy, to receive their education. Community members have the right to get the best service, which is fortunately free, but there is a long waitlist, and they have to be able to come to the hospital to access care. Those who can afford it have private sessions at home.

I bring up the wealth in next-door Israel and the inequities faced by Palestinians, and he responds, "I accept the culture of others, even my enemy. I can learn from them and apply that in Palestine."

He received training from a professor in Tel Aviv and is grateful for the experience in bringing this knowledge to Gaza.

In 2000, Moussa started a community rehabilitation program. Not everyone could access hospitals because of checkpoints dividing the Gaza Strip at the time. These checkpoints could result in journeys of several days, with people sleeping in their cars and unable to use the toilet. Though I remain stolid, my mouth drops open when he recalls a time when a checkpoint was closed and he went through the woods to provide community care and was shot at by soldiers. This is the level of dedication Moussa has to his people and profession. At the time, the community teams would work three days in a row and go home when the next team was able to relieve them, so service was never discontinued. Once access in and out for the country closed, these checkpoints were gone.

I ask Moussa to share what he loves most about his work. He initially wanted a good opportunity to work and make a living, but he soon began to focus on service, his responsibility towards his community, and the changes needed. Leaning back in his seat with contemplation and calm, he describes his prior motivation as selfish, and now, "I see others more than myself. Myself is reflected in others. You will find your happiness in their happiness. It's unfair to be happy when the people around you are sad and crying. It's not happiness. It's enjoying another's pain."

Sharing his hopes for occupational therapy in Palestine, Moussa gives a beautifully detailed response that also hits hard, reflecting the reality of life there. "If I live one year only, I want to see bachelor's and master's degrees in occupational therapy available in the Gaza Strip. If I live five years in addition to that, I would like to see an Arab-wide conference that Palestinians from both the West Bank and Gaza could access. If live ten years, I will develop a Palestinian occupational therapy model," what he calls "our identity, the doi [digital object identifier] of occupational therapy." He wants to be dean of the occupational therapy department as well. He laughs for the first time, knowing he should be considering retirement as he will be 65 by then. He started planning for retirement this year. Displaying some relief and contentment, he says he has shifted his plans and wants to be a journal reviewer in retirement. It will give him energy when he retires. A self-proclaimed, life-long learner, in retirement he wants to keep learning from occupational therapists worldwide.

He advises readers to add value and plant seeds no matter what we do: "Accept for others what you accept for yourself." He encourages us to find a way to push for positive changes and create a legacy. Research and publications are his legacies and added value. "Our life is a citation. Our ideas and values extend our life and legacy," he adds.

If he had a chance to do anything differently in his life, he wouldn't. We end our conversation by wishing each other *shukran* (thanks) and *salam* (peace), the few Arabic words I know. Smiling, pleased with the details he has shared with me, Moussa offers final words leaning into the screen, more animated than I have seen him in the past three and half hours: "Life is good and beautiful with peace. We are struggling for peace."

SUGGESTED NEXT STEPS

Reflection: Where and how do you notice occupational apartheid happening in your region?

Action: How are you planning to leave your legacy? Big or small, list your intentions.

Note: As of this publication, Moussa has successfully defended his dissertation and completed his PhD.

References

Abu Mostafa, M.K., Plastow, N.A., & Savin-Baden, M. (2023). "Participatory methods to develop health education for PW-SCI: Perspectives on occupational justice." *Canadian Journal of Occupational Therapy*, 90(1): 55–67, doi: 10.1177/00084174221116250.

Al Jazeera. (2022, August 5). A guide to the Gaza Strip. *Gaza News*. Al Jazeera. www.aljazeera.com/news/2021/3/14/a-guide-to-the-gaza-strip.

CEIC. (n.d.). *State of Palestine (West Bank and Gaza) median age: Gaza Strip*. www.ceicdata.com/en/palestinian-territory-occupied/vital-statistics/median-age-gaza-strip.

Humaid, M. (2022). The seven border crossings of Gaza. Israel–Palestine conflict. Al Jazeera. www.aljazeera.com/features/2022/6/15/the-seven-border-crossings-of-gaza.

Mostafa, M.A., Plastow, N.A., Savin-Baden, M., & Ayele, B. (2022) "The impact of an evidence-informed spinal cord injury activities of daily living education manual (SADL-eM): Protocol for a randomized controlled trial." *JMIR Research Protocols*, 11(7): e30611

Naser-Najjab, N. (2020). "Palestinian leadership and the contemporary significance of the First Intifada." *Race & Class*, 62(2): 61–79, https://doi.org/10.1177/0306396820946294.

Pappe, I. (2006). *The Ethnic Cleansing of Palestine*. London: Oneworld Publications.

United Nations. (n.d.). History of the Question of Palestine. www.un.org/unispal/history.

CHAPTER 3

PHILIPPINES: John Ray Lucas

While speaking with John, I hear birds chirping outside, elated and engaging with good energy, like him. He is wearing a deep blue polo shirt that is vivid among the lush green trees and sunlight shining through thick leaves reflected in the mirrors behind him. His clean-shaven face, short, dark black hair brushed to one side, and wide smile signals his excitement and preparedness for this interview.

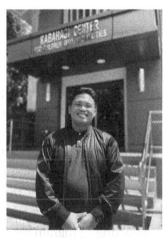

Figure 3.1: John standing in front of Kabahagi Center for Children with Disabilities

John Ray Lucas is a 38-year-old occupational therapist with many roles in Manila, Philippines. He has worked for a community-based, non-governmental organization (NGO), a pediatric clinic, and a school-based program, taught at a university, volunteered in disaster areas, and recently worked with his colleagues in an online political advocacy group for occupational therapists and students to represent a presidential candidate. He is currently a pediatric occupational therapist and program consultant for a government-led, community-based facility for parents and children with disabilities.

John has a bachelor's degree in occupational therapy and a master's degree in community development. This education, combined with his energy and enthusiasm, has led him to many unique opportunities. It seems natural for John to fall into leadership roles. When studying community development, his classmates were surprised that he knew how to facilitate groups while still a student. As an occupational therapist, he was trained in running groups and group dynamics, and he has combined his expertise in both fields in his work today.

Laughing, John tells me he became an occupational therapist by accident. He wanted to be a doctor and had to take pre-medical courses. Enrolling in occupational therapy courses without knowing anything about them, he learned more about himself in the process. Then, realizing he wanted to be part of a caring profession, he decided to no longer go to medical school because occupational therapy was right for him. With over ten years of experience as an occupational therapist working in many settings, he was even asked to consult for a film about an autistic child. Using his occupational therapy and advocacy experience, he explained to the actors and the director how society responds to autistic children and their families.

As a program consultant, John implements occupational therapy programs in institutions that do not currently have these services. Some of his past program development includes adding pediatric occupational therapy in a hospital, building sensory gyms, and starting a community-based rehabilitation program. He is currently supporting a program for adolescents with developmental disabilities transitioning to college to successfully obtain a degree. As in many Asian countries, education is highly valued, and a degree is meaningful. He's not afraid to take on new challenges and build programs from scratch. John's face lights up when he describes his work, and he keeps adding more details of his involvement. Each time he pauses, he adds another role he has taken on.

In the community-based rehabilitation (CBR) program, he co-initiated a pilot program to educate families, making the impact more long-term and sustainable. Here, children are not left to work alone with a therapist. Instead, parents and caregivers work in collaboration with them in every session. These facilities are closer to homes in rural areas than hospitals and most rehabilitation services, which tend to be in bigger cities. However, many families still have transportation issues. The cost of transportation can be prohibitive, so the CBR facility assists with paying for and arranging transportation. In addition, the CBR program is funded by the government, making all services free while providing payment to therapists.

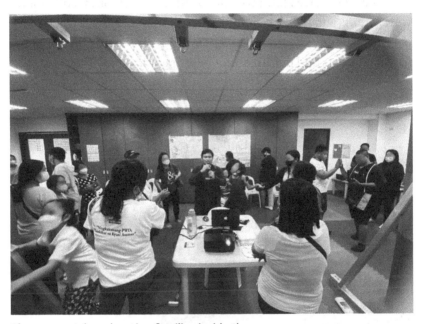

Figure 3.2: John educating families inside the community-based rehabilitation program

John and his team use social media to reach these communities for advertising services, educational events, and webinars. In addition, they developed a parent support group to mobilize parents to support other parents of disabled children. There are almost 200 members in this group, and they also help spread the word about occupational therapy services to the local community. His goal is to empower the community to provide long-term, sustainable care, as there are not enough occupational therapists to support all the children and families who could benefit from services.

He is also a mentor for occupational therapy students training in Visayas and Mindanao, areas with limited services and access. Manila, the most densely populated city in the world, is located on the largest island in the country, Luzon. People in the capital city of Manila tend to receive better-quality care, which is why John is committed to ensuring best practices for people outside Manila and in remote regions. Some have to commute an hour to the nearest city to access telehealth appointments if they don't have the internet at home. The lack of access drives John to work with new therapists, collaborate with parents and the community, and continue care, even when occupational therapy is hard to reach. Done right, occupational therapy fits all contexts and cultures and meets people where they are.

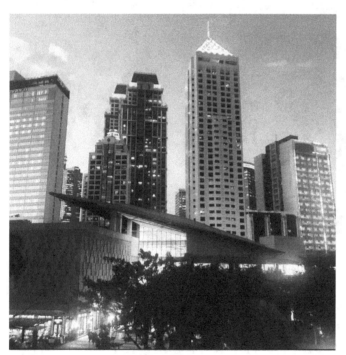

Figure 3.3: The Makati skyline taken from John's phone

Working with a developmental pediatrician, who also happens to be an occupational therapist, John ensures that rural health services are as good as those available in the city. The hard-to-reach areas typically don't have access to physicians and occupational therapy, so with help from a developmental pediatrician to send referrals, they offer therapy services virtually.

Recently, John supported a campaign for a presidential candidate. In just three days, he and his team mobilized almost 1000 occupational therapy students and professionals, a significant portion of the nearly 4500 occupational therapists in the country. This recent election ignited a spark within many occupational therapists and students in the country, who recognized that professional responsibilities go beyond the immediate services we deliver and include eliminating barriers to appropriate care, reducing health and resource inequities, and increasing access to care. The group he started is raising awareness, advocating for compassionate leadership, and is continuing to grow.

In practice, part of John's political advocacy includes teaching the families he works with about their voting right, how they can exercise that right, and where to get accurate information on candidates and issues on the ballot. He has also been helping his wider community become more aware of how politics impacts health services, depending on who is in office. Ensuring that regardless of income, everyone can access quality care is justice. Unfortunately, many people in the Philippines cannot afford services because they are too expensive. Through community organizing activities, John wants to make the government sectors aware of rehabilitation services so they can create more occupational, physical, and speech therapy positions.

He has seen this in action. The CBR program he works in was started because the incumbent mayor prioritized helping people with disabilities and hiring allied health professionals. With government and multi-sectoral support, these programs can be sustainable, and John wants to see this happen at higher levels of government. This isn't unique to the Philippines. Wherever we are in the world, the government influences healthcare services and who can access them.

John firmly believes that occupational therapy is political. Occupational therapists can make collaborative decisions with the family and the team, and this can help transfer power to the people so that they can make changes for themselves, their families, and their communities. Healthcare in the Philippines, including therapy services, is expensive, and, if subsidized by the government, more people would be able to access services. Only the privileged few who can afford it can access care around the country. As a profession, politics affects our wages and where we can practice. There is no way to remove politics from the occupational context as it is ingrained in everything.

Occupational therapy textbooks in the Philippines have a Western lens, so he has adapted what he learned in practice for the contexts in which he works. Though the Philippines has been historically influenced by colonization by Spain and later the United States, Filipino culture remains communal and family-oriented, with family and community members helping each other rather than prioritizing independence. These values make occupational priorities different from Western ones. John teaches his students to challenge what they learn if it doesn't fit the needs of the people with whom they work. The most effective way he has found is to have students spend time in the areas they are not from, regularly working in rural areas and frequently returning to get to know the people and regions. He teaches students to respect local culture and use their existing resources, instead of changing their daily practices. For instance, access to adaptive equipment and specialized tools for pediatric interventions is difficult and cost prohibitive. So, they work with items found inside the home. The solutions come from the people with whom they work, while the occupational therapists help facilitate rather than dictate goals and interventions.

I ask John how he explains occupational therapy to children and families. He doesn't have an elevator pitch, always keeping his explanation simple while changing it depending on the person and context, including using the local language when talking to community members. Using the everyday language of the families he works with, rather than unnecessary jargon, he focuses on sharing examples that fit into their daily lives. Even though various languages and dialects are spoken throughout the country, English is primarily used in practice.

John is from Manila, and sometimes travels to rural areas for work. His community development education has helped him significantly in immersing himself in the community to be more effective. He's lived and worked with Indigenous groups, the urban poor, and victims of disasters in relocation sites. He focuses on indigenizing interventions within the local culture, teaching students to use the things people have and use in their homes instead of introducing new adaptive equipment, because many cannot afford or access this. Even with telehealth, he first checks what people have at home and works with what they have. "We don't want to change their practice, just adapt and then use their existing assets. It's very important you're not teaching them to live life the way that you do. You're meeting them where they are," he urges. Humility translates to anywhere in the world, especially when working with people with different life experiences from our own. We are not experts; we are there to listen and learn.

One of the biggest challenges John faces is shifting mindsets to empower people. Many people don't know what occupational therapy is, while some don't think they need occupational therapy, or they don't trust occupational therapists because they aren't from their village. A survey he and his colleagues completed with rural communities revealed that one of the most significant barriers to accepting services was they could not prioritize it because of work. Going to a facility to receive occupational therapy services or working on home programs interferes with making a living to support themselves and their families. Many of the parents he works with have partners working overseas, so they cannot afford to take time off of work and do not have support at home to help continue with therapy recommendations.

Much of John's work is advocacy based. He works with families to gain access to a Person with Disability Card (PWD). Many parents don't realize they can apply for the card if their children are disabled. The card provides discounts on medical expenses, food, transportation, and recreation. It is a formal identification and gives legitimacy to a disability identity. He asserts, "When you know your rights, you're able to advocate for your rights." Occupational justice is about ensuring access. He sees occupational therapy as having a role in every aspect of society, in every context. He even collaborated with architects to increase their awareness of inclusive design. There are accessibility laws in place, but they are poorly implemented. For example, stair heights and ramps are not often accessible.

When asked what he loves most about his work, John pauses, looking into the distance, "It's that good feeling that you get when you can help people." He displays a huge teeth-bearing smile, and it's clear that he loves what he does. His roles involve creating networks and community, which he beams about when discussing them. He enjoys traveling and relishes work-related travel to meet with physicians, occupational therapists, and other professionals he works with online. This work energizes him, and he finds it sustainable, affording him occupational balance. Chuckling, he knows he's overly involved professionally, but he makes time to run daily, do CrossFit, and write about his work.

There are many ways that John has been able to use his occupational therapy experience. A regular volunteer, he stepped up to help after Super Typhoon Yolanda, one of the deadliest typhoons in the Philippines that resulted in the evacuation of over five million people. Initially, he was volunteering at the air force base, managing the graveyard shift of the feeding program. Coming in every day after work and full days on his days off, feeding survivors and soldiers, he made sandwiches, prepped ingredients, delivered food, washed dishes, cleaned, and oriented new volunteers. With limited supplies, he had to be creative with what was available, making eggs in as many ways as he knew how—boiled, fried, omelets, and frittatas—always focused on fostering a supportive environment that would comfort survivors of a traumatic event with a long, arduous journey ahead.

He recalls meeting a group of men who had waited days to be evacuated with only bottled water and biscuits. Like the rest of the evacuees, they expressed gratitude for the warm food and care volunteers like John provided. Afterward, he flew to a hard-hit region where there were many casualties and destroyed homes to initiate a feeding program, which made a significant impact on locally affected residents during a devastating time.

John appreciates how flexible the profession of occupational therapy is. It is adaptable and dynamic and adjusts to any person, setting, place, or context. Occupational therapy practice is a representation of people. He believes in respecting traditions. Case studies and teachings in textbooks are not always representative; we should "meet people where they are rather than having them conform to our idea of what they're supposed to be doing."

Much of occupational therapy practice in the Philippines is focused on pediatrics and hospital settings. John innovates programs to get therapists where they are most needed and offers them a chance to learn and grow. He is excited for occupational therapy in the Philippines to broaden practice areas, create more innovative programs to explore new niches, and go beyond a medical focus into social and rights-based concerns. John hopes for occupational therapy in the Philippines to include more occupational therapists in all provinces. In addition, there are many Philippine-trained occupational therapists who practice abroad, and he hopes they will return to give back to their home communities.

He dreams of having occupational therapists involved in policy-making at all levels, from local to global, to advocate for disability inclusion and services. Policy is how changes are enacted, and his political advocacy is apparent with his election-mobilizing efforts. For the profession to be sustainable, occupational therapists should collaborate globally to share best practices and learn from each other.

John's advice for readers is to listen to people and empathize with them. That is the first step in understanding and building a relationship. First, we have to know ourselves. Next, build relationships with clients, colleagues, the community, and anyone we work with. Good communication in fostering a relationship is listening—and this is universal advice for being a good person or professional.

As we wrap up the conversation, John thanks me for the chat and shares that he has been sad the past few days because of the election results, and this conversation has given him the strength to keep pushing for a better world. The smile on his face is still there, but sadness creeps into his eyes. His hope for a better future in the Philippines keeps him going, but it's not easy to persist. I'm reminded of Leni Robredo's words during her concession speech in the 2022 Philippine presidential election:

What I've learned from difficult situations is that healing does not come while you're sulking on your own. It comes when you start focusing on other people... Allow yourself to cry, but when you're ready to wipe away your tears, prepare yourself, strengthen your heart because we have work to do. (Wee & Elemia, 2022)

SUGGESTED NEXT STEPS

Reflection: How do you think occupational therapy is political? In what areas should the profession be more politically involved?

Action: In what ways will you get involved in political advocacy?

References

Wee, S.-L. & Elemia, C. (2022). "Robredo admits defeat in Philippine presidential election." New York Times. www.nytimes.com/2022/05/13/world/asia/robredo-philippine-election.html.

CHAPTER 4

NEPAL: Dorothy Das Pariyar

On a Wednesday evening after work, Dorothy calls in from her mobile phone. It's 6am for me in San Francisco. I can see her face surrounded by long, black wavy hair parted in the middle, wearing what appears to be a light blue kurta from the visible collar and a deep peach-colored wall behind her in her home in Pokhara, Nepal. With a smile, she tells me she is nervous.

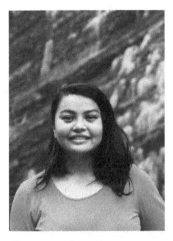

Figure 4.1: Dorothy standing in front of a steep hillside waterfall

Dorothy Das Pariyar is a young occupational therapist with three years of clinical experience after getting her bachelor's degree from Indore, India.

She is curious about the book and my experiences, asking with genuine interest about the book's purpose before we begin the interview. I tell her that although occupational therapy is practiced worldwide and I live in a culturally diverse country, I didn't experience adequate global representation in occupational therapy education. Over 12 years later, access to occupational therapy research and practice globally is still limited. In fact, despite my heritage, I didn't meet any South Asian occupational therapists until a couple of years ago. I hope this book will end up in programs worldwide so people can learn about the profession from different perspectives, realizing there are many ways to do, be, and practice occupational therapy. We should learn about occupational therapies and stories that represent more of the world.

Though much of occupational therapy education worldwide is from Western texts, using a Western lens, every country has its cultures and ways of doing. I want to give people a window into how occupational therapy is different and similar in various countries. Dorothy resonates with this, recalling that her studies in India did not include occupational therapy from India or Nepal. Significant adapting was required to fit what she learned into Nepali contexts, including little to no access to new adaptive technology and devices.

Nepal has no occupational therapy schools, so I am curious as to how Dorothy decided to become an occupational therapist. Her father's friend, a physician in England, suggested that Dorothy might be interested in the profession because his daughter was an occupational therapist. Though she hadn't known about the profession until her father mentioned it, Dorothy was always interested in working in healthcare. She got to stay at a facility in Surkhet, Nepal, for five days where an occupational therapist from England was working in neuro rehabilitation, something she was unfamiliar with. In awe, she speaks about the impact of observing therapy sessions. She felt a strong connection to the work, and seeing someone come from abroad to serve Nepali people called her to become an occupational therapist to work within her own community.

Dorothy and her family invested in her future. She moved to India for high school to access better education and lived in an all-girls hostel. Calling her parents in Nepal was difficult and infrequent because she could only have short five- to ten-minute phone conversations, with one shared phone for all the residents. Though it was a challenge for her, this experience prepared her to live in India for four and a half years for occupational therapy education and training.

Green Pastures Hospital in Pokhara, Nepal, is celebrating 70 years of service this year. It is the first facility in Nepal to have an occupational therapist. The hospital was established to provide services for people affected by leprosy and later became a full-service rehabilitation hospital, including palliative care. It is where three of the ten occupational therapists in the country work. Only eight of the ten currently practice. Dorothy covers inpatient and outpatient services here. When she joined in 2019, there were no occupational therapists, only occupational therapy assistants. Occupational therapy assistants have been at this hospital for over three decades. Occupational therapists have worked in the hospital but have since left to further their education and either remained abroad or moved to different roles outside the hospital.

Lyndal Henry, a volunteer from Aotearoa New Zealand, brought occupational therapy to Nepal in 1985 (Association of Nepal's Occupational Therapists, n.d.). She came to Green Pastures Hospital to teach people with leprosy how to save their hands, to limit deformities and ulcers, and to offer independence. Vocational training, such as tailoring and candle making, allowed patients to return home and support their families financially. In addition, she addressed the stigma of being accepted back into communities when returning home.

Thirty-seven years after Lyndal Henry brought occupational therapy to Nepal, there are only ten occupational therapists and eleven occupational therapy assistants, though one recently retired. When Dorothy went to India for her occupational therapy education, there were only four occupational therapists in Nepal. However, there has been significant professional growth in the past few years. Dorothy was fortunate that her hospital sponsored her education abroad. Since she joined, two additional occupational therapists have been sponsored to gain their education abroad and return to the hospital to practice.

It's rare for a facility to sponsor education. People have to fund their own international occupational therapy education, which is expensive. It is common to leave the country for education, stay abroad, and not bring the profession back home. There are more work opportunities and higher salaries abroad for people to send money back home. Still, Dorothy wants to work on promoting the profession locally. She is hopeful that her friend, an occupational therapist running for Miss Nepal, might bring a national spotlight to the profession. She is one of the top 24 finalists and works with children in Kathmandu.

The country's occupational therapists meet every six months to discuss promoting the profession and working on government recognition. Until very recently, it was not a registered profession, meaning anyone could claim to be an occupational therapist with or without training and formal education. The Association of Nepal's Occupational Therapists just became registered with the Nepal Health Professional Council, a big step toward national recognition and setting standards. Some clinics and hospitals claim to offer occupational therapy but do not have any trained occupational therapists on staff. Establishing occupational therapy with the government would set specific standards and professional boundaries to prevent this from happening. There is a misunderstanding that anyone can be an occupational therapist. Until there are more qualified occupational therapists that the government fully recognizes, professional growth will continue to be stunted.

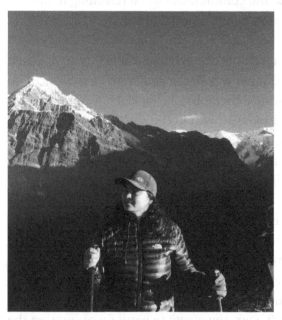

Figure 4.2: Dorothy standing in front of large snow-capped mountains holding walking sticks

Nepal is home to सगरमाथा (*Sagarmatha*), also known as Mount Everest, the tallest mountain in the world above sea level. The city of Pokhara is located in the hilly Pokhara Valley. It is the second most populated city in Nepal after Kathmandu, the capital. People from surrounding areas come to Green Pastures for care. Patients that leave the hospital requiring a wheelchair for mobility may not have access in their homes or hometowns. Many live in hilly areas, making mobility challenging. Many homes have steps and cannot accommodate ramps, so there is no accessibility for people with mobility issues. They might have to be carried down the stairs to get into a vehicle for medical appointments. Space in homes can be limited, making it impossible to turn a wheelchair indoors. Home visits are not possible except for palliative care, because of limited staffing. However, there was a time when home visits for people with spinal cord injuries (SCI) were happening. The hospital is trying to restart this program.

In Dorothy's region, there is a trend among poor people for acquiring spinal cord injuries, as their work is riskier. Work may involve construction or climbing trees, resulting in falls and SCIs. Older people who have had a stroke were often engaged in farming and may be unable to return to work. Some change their profession and learn new skills that they can complete to earn an income. Many people have had to leave their rural communities and move into the city because it is more accessible and they can find more accommodating work. Part of Dorothy's role is working with newly disabled people to find new careers, navigate role changes at home, and reintegrate into their community. Not everyone is ready. When patients return to the hospital for follow-up or additional care, they are more willing to accept the changes to their life. The hospital has two peer counselors who are wheelchair users. One works in the occupational therapy department to support and motivate patients to reach their goals.

The minimum stay at Green Pastures is 14 days and averages between 14 and 21 days, with a required follow-up stay of one week for additional education. Occasionally, long-term patients stay for three to four months due to grade four pressure sores, common with SCIs. Depression and lack of engagement with paid work, family responsibilities, and community involvement often result in decreased motivation to follow through with rehabilitation training to prevent pressure sores. They have weekly interdisciplinary meetings to discuss all concerns, including socioeconomic factors. Outpatient visits are typically from nearby patients who come once or twice weekly for follow-up after discharge. Telehealth is also an option.

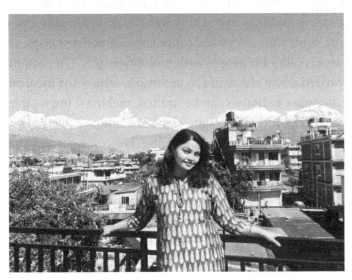

Figure 4.3: Dorothy standing against a balcony in a residential neighborhood in Pokhara, with snow-capped mountains in the distance

Dorothy speaks Nepali, Hindi, and English. Nepali is predominantly spoken while working, though some people are comfortable with English. पेशा (*pesha*) is occupation in Nepali, though it describes work. When explaining to patients and family, Dorothy prefers to use the English word occupation as there is no Nepali word or phrase to capture an accurate translation. She tries to promote functional independence, a concept often easier to accept for younger generations than older ones. In Nepali culture, like many South Asian cultures, there is an expectation that younger family members will care for older, ill, and disabled family members. The desire to be independent depends on the person, generation, and culture. She stresses that it is important to remain respectful of people's wants and traditions regardless of their preferences. Though more women are going to school and having careers, there is often no one at home to take care of older family members, making it a necessary conversation to have with patients and their families.

No occupational therapists work in psychiatry, though Dorothy's work in the hospital involves psychosocial factors and concerns. There are a lot of challenges and opportunities for education and advocacy. She provides counseling for grieving losses and adapting to new roles and circumstances.

"The thing that I love about my profession is to see the smile when they are able to do something that they were not able to do, and they're very happy," Dorothy shares while touching her heart. She values the impact she makes on families, not just individuals. Families are heavily involved in the rehabilitation process. An adult family member or caregiver must stay with patients during admission, attend therapy sessions, and eventually support the person at home. Depending on the needs of the patient and the involvement of the family or caregiver, nursing support is decreased during their stay. Family involvement often helps patients to be more motivated to work with therapists and treatment as they may want to go home and be with family instead of being at the hospital. Having family stay can make patients feel more comfortable. At the same time, the family or caregiver will better understand the rehabilitation process.

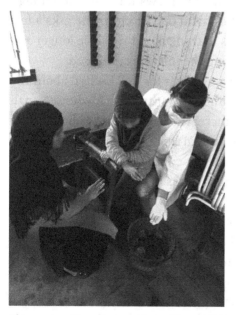

Figure 4.4: Dorothy working with a child and parent in the hospital

Ninety minutes into our conversation Dorothy's power goes out. Calling in from her mobile phone, she can continue the conversation, her face lit up by the screen alone. I can still see her facial expressions. It's common for the power to go out in storms, though it wasn't raining today and she isn't sure why the power went out. A minor setback, but we continue.

Her Indian training was different. In the acute care hospital setting in India, she worked with patients and did not have much opportunity to interact with their families, which is an essential part of her work now in the rehabilitation hospital in Nepal. This makes me reflect on the patient-centered care I was taught to practice in the United States, which involves the person, rarely their family, and never the community. It is necessary to consider families when treating the person, especially when living in multi-generational households is the norm. Dorothy is practicing patient- and family-centered care to ensure the patient can return home successfully with the family support they need.

Dorothy is insecure about her responses to the final question about her hopes for global occupational therapy. She is concerned she is "representing Nepal," so she doesn't want to "miss anything." She pauses to think, putting her hand on her chin. She asks a few clarifying questions and decides to think about it a little longer and get back to me later with anything she might have missed.

I ask Dorothy if she has any questions for me. Excited about the opportunity, she jumps right in. She wants to know how Nepali occupational therapists might increase their knowledge base with a limited number of senior occupational therapists, all with bachelor's degrees. I offer to connect her and her colleagues with occupational therapists in countries with similar issues in establishing themselves and growing.

Curious about my education, as I have a master's degree in occupational therapy, she wants to know if it would be helpful for her also to get a master's. She wants to further her studies and bring new practices back home. I offer a few suggestions, including connecting with occupational therapists in different parts of the world and practicing abroad. It's expensive and another degree does not always mean she will be able to apply what she learns back home. Dorothy wants to connect with occupational therapists abroad and agrees. The head of her department mentioned something similar; there are many ways to get further education and experience, and there's no one path. It's best to explore options and figure out what is best for you.

Fifteen minutes later, the power comes back on and I can see Dorothy and the colorful wall behind her again. We are at the end of the interview, and Dorothy shares her gratitude for being included in the book and being able to represent Nepal. She offers an open invitation to support me with anything I need help with. I offer thanks to Dorothy in Nepali, *dhanyabaad*, a word I am familiar with because it is similar in Hindi.

SUGGESTED NEXT STEPS

Reflection: How valued is community or family involvement in your practice?

Action: What can you do to incorporate more family- or community-based care?

References

Association of Nepal's Occupational Therapists. (n.d.). When we started. https://anotnepal.wordpress.com/when-we-started.

CHAPTER 5

GHANA: Ann Sena Fordie

Ann Sena Fordie has been an occupational therapist in Accra, Ghana, for six years. She assumes many roles, including head of the occupational therapy department at Pantang Hospital, Clinical Director of Sena Pediatric Therapy, her namesake, and President of the Occupational Therapy Association of Ghana. The first of four siblings, she's used to being like a second mother and taking care of her younger siblings, so she has always loved working with children and finds herself in roles where she is leading and caring for people.

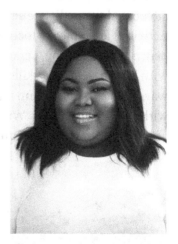

Figure 5.1: Close-up photo of Ann smiling

I first heard Ann speak on the *OT & Chill* podcast and was compelled to reach out and connect with her. Kwaku Agyemang, the host of the show, is also Ghanian and works as an occupational therapist in the United Kingdom (UK). In that episode, they discussed occupational therapy in Ghana and the stigma around mental illness. When someone has a mental illness, the cultural perception often is that they are condemned and cannot do anything for themselves. It's much harder for people to recognize that improving function and social integration are possible with a mental illness than with a physical one. There's less hope.

The stigma of mental illness negatively impacts all areas of life,

occupations especially. An example Ann shared of the profound misunderstanding and shame is if it's found that someone in the family
has a mental illness, a prospective marriage might be called off. Education is ongoing as the stigma is strong. Younger generations have a
better understanding, which brings her some hope. Ann, along with
other mental health advocates, is changing the narrative through
education, outreach, and empowering people with mental illness to
overcome challenges, do the things they want, and participate in
society and life as fully as anyone else.

At Pantang Hospital, named after a nearby village, Ann works
in adult and pediatric mental health. Originally serving adults, she
advocated for pediatric services and helped develop that program.
Activities are typically focused on vocations like basket weaving, car-
pentry, dressmaking, ceramics, and gardening. Some help patients
with income-earning skills, though most are for finding meaningful
ways to occupy time. Ann is proud of what they have been able to do
with limited resources. Wishing they had access to more, activities
are limited to what they can obtain.

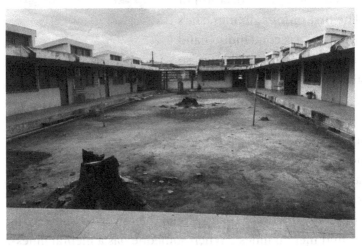

Figure 5.2: Outdoor occupational therapy group
activity space at Pantang Hospital

After discharge, they aim for weekly reviews. There aren't sufficient
resources for home visits, so follow-up typically occurs over the

phone or via video calls. A nearby community occupational therapist is set up for home visits and works with discharged patients in her area to check and report on their progress when needed. Another local hospital is set up for community visits, but clients must pay for services there. Only those who can afford it have access to these services.

Sena Pediatric Therapy is the first non-governmental organization in Ghana to offer occupational, speech, and physical therapies. Ann is humble, so I have to point out that she has created a first-of-its-kind pediatric therapy facility and insist she celebrates this accomplishment. They support children and work towards inclusive education in the country. It's easier for her to convince parents of the benefits of occupational therapy at Sena Pediatric Therapy than in mental health settings. Parents are more inclined to invest in and pay for services to support their children with improving handwriting, communication, social interactions, cognitive skills, and other areas that occupational therapy typically addresses.

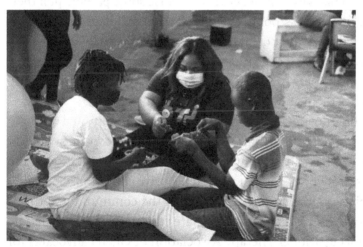

Figure 5.3: Ann working with an older child and parent

Therapy services occur once or twice a week, so they work with children, their families, and caregivers to continue with occupational therapy plans outside the clinic and improve outcomes. They also work with teachers, write reports, and develop individualized educational plans for caregivers and teachers to work with children at school. The more people involved in the child's goals, the more improvement there will be. Remote teacher training is another method they use to stay updated on what happens at school. By empowering family members and people in the community, the work continues even in places where families can't access the clinic and therapists can't reach families.

Ann shares painful stories of families hiding children or keeping them locked away because they don't believe they can participate in school and society. They don't have hope and don't see the point of therapy. Sena's mission is to empower parents and show them that disabled children can attend school and learn to care for themselves. This requires access to supportive services early in life.

Education is a big part of their work to reach out to families that don't know about occupational therapy or don't have any hope that it can help their children. Ann goes to local schools to train and educate community members by attending parent–teacher association meetings. This is even more critical because some parents pull their children out of classrooms when a disabled child enrolls. There is a false belief that their child might catch what a disabled child has. Ann provides critical education to debunk these harmful myths. She spends time helping parents understand how their children can learn, and teaches them about inclusive education.

Her clinic does many school visits in the community and throughout the country on virtual platforms. They were even invited to speak to teachers and parents in Nigeria. Soon she will be going to churches to advocate for therapy and inclusive education. Ghanaians are religious, and churches are pillars of the community, so this is an effective way to build trust and share education and information.

The Occupational Therapy Association of Ghana advocates for occupational therapy in the country by providing support to occupational therapy professionals, accrediting courses, and offering professional development and continuing education opportunities. As the President of the Association, Ann's primary role is to advocate for the profession and service users. Her role includes ensuring that members have employment opportunities in various settings and are paid a good salary. The Ministry of Education invited her to put together a policy for inclusive education in Ghana. This is another thing she doesn't want to brag about, but, I insist, is a big deal. As President of the Association, she represents the profession at meetings and conferences. She is also responsible for organizing continuing education for members, including finding speakers.

The Association has a committee for researching and developing contextually relevant practices. Most occupational therapy knowledge is borrowed from Western parts of the world. The research committee is working on a document describing Ghanaian occupational therapy's scope of practice. With only 114 occupational therapy professionals in the country, only a few people are involved in this extensive work. Still, outreach and advocacy are a focus, and Ann puts in significant time and effort in all of these areas.

Ann was in the first cohort of occupational therapists to study in Ghana. After completing high school, a written examination determines your field of study for university. Unfamiliar with occupational therapy, Ann wanted to study medicine or pharmacy. After taking the exam, she did not qualify for medical school and was assigned a course in occupational therapy instead. Her father was living in the United States (US) at the time and looked into this career choice. He thought it would be a viable and engaging profession, offering her a good salary. At the time, Ann considered it an opportunity to return to her dream of becoming a doctor through a graduate entry medical program.

The first year of studies was very challenging and frustrating. Ann couldn't even explain what she was studying to her friends because she didn't understand the profession herself. Her fieldwork placements were with various clinicians, not occupational therapists. Some would fall under nursing or medicine, and they didn't know what occupational therapy was. Nevertheless, Ann kept pushing forward because she ultimately wanted to pursue medicine.

It was in her third year that it all came together. She had an opportunity to travel to the UK for a placement as part of an exchange program. Here she learned under occupational therapists and understood what occupational therapy was and what occupational therapists do. Loving what she saw, she became passionate about occupational therapy. Her face brightens as she relives the joy she then found. The ideas about what she wanted to bring back to Ghana filled her head—how she could change things, what she could do, and the way she could help her community.

A Ghanaian occupational therapist, Dr. Peter Ndaa, brought occupational therapy to Ghana. He was working in a Ghanaian facility with an occupational therapist in the mental health system. After the therapist retired, there was no occupational therapist to replace the position, so he was asked to go to the UK to study occupational therapy and manage the department when he returned. At the time, there were no occupational therapy programs in Ghana, so he completed his master's degree abroad. Realizing this would eventually be a problem again, he helped create an occupational therapy program in Ghana in 2012. Eighteen students, including Ann, were part of the inaugural class. A diploma program is available in the country for occupational therapy assistants, and a bachelor's in occupational therapy at the University of Ghana. For a master's degree or PhD, occupational therapists must leave the country to study.

Her education was based on Western occupational therapy. The education program has likely improved since Ann's inaugural class, so she can't speak about its current state. Adaptations have since been made for education to be more relevant to the Ghanaian context. She and her classmates were guinea pigs, learning from Western textbooks not made for the African context, with methods that did not apply to the people of Ghana. While in the UK, Ann was taught to have someone make a cup of tea to assess their skills. Taking tea is not common in Ghanaian culture. Hence, a common adaptation is to make a simple dish of gari made with cassava roots. Like Ann, her classmates had to adapt their learning to suit the local culture and context.

Occupational therapy licensing is with the Allied Health Professions Council, part of the Ministry of Health in Ghana. The government formally recognizes the profession, and there are systems for government health programs with occupational therapists included. Recognition, legitimacy, and funding from the government are critical to getting appropriate services to people who need them. Mental health is occupational therapy's primary function in Ghana. It has been challenging to include occupational therapy in other settings like physical disabilities, neurology, and pediatrics.

There are currently 62 occupational therapists in Ghana and 52 occupational therapy assistants, totaling 114 occupational therapy practitioners in the country. Considering the first cohort of occupational therapists graduated only six years ago and locally trained Ghanaians can find higher salaries and better-resourced institutions abroad, these are solid numbers. From Ghana, it's easy to find the wages occupational therapists make abroad and compare them to what they are making working in the same profession. For those who have studied abroad for their master's or PhD, it is tempting not to return when they receive offers for jobs in those countries. Many Ghanaian occupational therapists are practicing in the UK, US, Canada, and Australia.

Ann chose to stay in Ghana to better establish occupational therapy in her home country. She loves her home and is putting all her energy into improving access to services, like the many others who have chosen to stay. Physical therapy is well known, but occupational therapy is still struggling to find its place in Ghana. For occupational therapy to grow, she recognizes that it must be in all spaces.

Ann actively encourages colleagues to consider government roles in parliament or other prominent positions to advocate for professional and healthcare needs. Occupational therapists in local government positions increase visibility for the profession and create more opportunities. To promote occupational therapy and rehabilitation in general, Ann plans to enter politics in a few years. Recognizing the government's power to make health policies, she wants occupational therapy not just to have a seat at the table but also to dominate those spaces. The profession is over 100 years old, yet we have been "too dormant...we should be on everyone's lips, we should be in beauty pageants, we should be in government positions, we should be in the UN, we should be in politics," she proclaims. Nothing is going to happen if we stay in our comfort zones. Ann is a compelling leader and confident speaker. I can't help but see her realizing her dreams.

Ga, Avatime, and English are the languages Ann primarily speaks, though she understands many more. English is the most common language spoken with clients, then Twi. The Association hired a linguist to help capture a good description of occupational therapy because the direct translation of occupation is job, which is inadequate. Therapy to help you function is what they came up with, which in Twi is *ahokeka mu apomhwe*.

In the middle of this discussion, Ann loses connection for a few minutes and returns. With her hair in a high half-ponytail, Ann is calling in on her phone with a bright white and lime green wall behind her and a tall palm tree peeking through the window at the back as she returns.

In Accra, the capital city and Ann's home, about 70 percent of the people receiving occupational therapy are local. However, some come from far away for therapy services. Recently, a family came from Benin looking for services for their child, which speaks to the reach of education and advocacy that Ann has been putting effort into.

There is national health insurance in Ghana, but that only covers simple medical procedures and essential medication. It does not cover rehabilitation. Funding for occupational therapy services is the most significant barrier to access. Government services are relatively inexpensive at about 65 cedis per session. Still, these are not one-time appointments and people need to be seen multiple times for benefit. One occupational therapy appointment might cost twice or more what a person is used to spending on an average day. Transportation is also an issue. There are cases where an organization can cover care, but the family does not have transportation, so they cannot access the service.

Understanding what occupational therapy does is another problem. Some physicians don't refer to the service despite its benefit to a patient because they are not aware of what an occupational therapist is and what they can offer families. Some people might stop services because they don't think they need them. It is challenging to meet the needs of everyone who could benefit from occupational therapy services. There is one occupational therapy practitioner for every 250,000 people. There's a growing need for occupational therapy, and Ann is working with the local community to fill it.

The roots of occupational therapy in Ghana are in mental health, as that is the original model brought to the country. Pediatrics is relatively new, though growing. It tends to be offered as a private service, making it costly and difficult for the average family to access. However, there is a new pediatrician in Ghana who was trained abroad and she has been diagnosing autism, cerebral palsy, and other conditions that should be addressed early in life. She is familiar with occupational therapy and has been educating parents about services and referring them. Currently, services for disabled children resemble respite care for parents to be able to go to work. Ann is hoping to make therapy a priority.

Accra is a colorful and bustling city. Ann says Ghanaian people like to wear African prints, as I notice her in a traditional dress with colors of red, brown, yellow, and occasional ocean blue emerging on the screen. Locals are hospitable, respectful, and have much pride in their culture. It's very sunny; "expect nothing but warm temperature," she says to me, as I wear a dark sweatshirt with a sweater on my lap to keep warm. If I visit, Ann insists, I'd have the best fun of my life. Ghanaians are happy and make the best out of every situation.

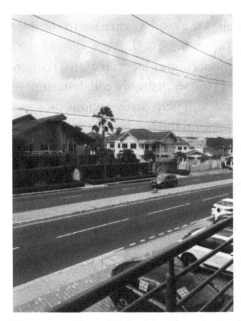

Figure 5.4: The neighborhood near Ann's clinic

The concept of independence, a common goal in occupational therapy, is "dicey," as Ghana is a communal society where people are used to helping each other. Ann shares an example of a relative having a stroke and the entire community coming together to care for them. She describes "communal love" and care as wanting to do everything for someone with an illness, injury, or disability. As an occupational therapist, she tries to help patients, family members, and caregivers understand that they could be at work making money if the person could have some independence in caring for themselves. Some are persuaded by this and open to therapy. But, in other cases, people feel indebted to the person who helped them and believe it is their time to reciprocate, sacrificing their income and livelihoods. There is a deep sense of duty and care for each other, even for people who are not related.

Ann wants to be able to walk into any room, introduce herself as an occupational therapist, and have everyone know what she does and rush to use her services when needed. Occupational therapists should be essential healthcare team members who receive referrals like other well-known and understood services. If more than one university offers occupational therapy courses, the therapist count could increase in the country, allowing more Ghanaians to consider pursuing and advancing the profession.

DisruptOT inspires global connections for occupational therapy professionals and students, and Ann wants more collaboration—a common platform to share ideas will help many regions progress in the profession together. At present, the barriers for people from low-income countries to study abroad in Western and other wealthy countries are too great, and it's too expensive to access education if programs don't exist in their regions. A global perspective would increase critical thinking and actions on access and reducing barriers. As it is, people are leaving Ghana for education and not returning to bring the profession back home.

Ann wants occupational therapists to be involved with disability policies and create a Ghanaian or African scope of occupational therapy practice that is not Western-directed. More textbooks from the African continent will meet the needs of the African context and support people in the diaspora to receive better and more culturally relevant care.

Ann would like a mentorship program for countries newer to the profession to gain more confidence and stability. Ideally, a free global network of mentors would be available to support lower- and middle-income countries. With an average occupational therapist's salary of 3000 cedis a month—well above the country's average salary—it's not feasible to pay for mentorship services. Currently, all programs to support occupational therapy professionals in Ghana are free because the Association wants everyone to have access and build and improve their skills. It is more concerned with developing effective, confident clinicians able to advocate for themselves than trying to make money as an association—something more national associations should be in favor of.

This is why I started an ongoing global partnership program and hope to someday create a traveling practitioner program through DisruptOT. The partnership network started with occupational therapists in Bangladesh connecting with other therapists globally after learning about barriers and challenges caused by the COVID-19 pandemic. The program is free to participate in, and people are paired based on their area of practice. It's more than mentorship; it's a partnership, as they learn from each other. If we wait for large organizations to build these programs, we will just be waiting around forever. Individuals like Ann and grassroots organizations like DisruptOT recognize the gaps and are working immediately to fill them.

Ann has several resources that have helped her learn and build her confidence. Recordings from the 2021 DisruptOT Community Summit, in which Ann speaks about the benefits of having a community for occupational therapy to share ideas, have valuable resources, be inspired, build confidence, and feel connected, are available on the DisruptOT YouTube channel. She listens to several podcasts to learn about occupational therapy practice: *OT Flourish*, *OT Potential*, *OT & Chill*, and the YouTube channel for LovelyyOT, by Nancy Yamoah, who also shares Ghanaian heritage.

Ann's advice for readers is to listen to clients and plan from a holistic point of view. She wants us to be proud of our profession and care for ourselves; otherwise, losing hope and leaving the profession can be easy. We should dominate spaces and advocate for the profession—make noise about occupational therapy and be assertive!

Now that you have read Ann's story, please take some time to think about occupational therapy in your context. You are invited to have a discussion with peers.

SUGGESTED NEXT STEPS

Reflection: In what ways can occupational therapy dominate spaces? What spaces? How?

Action: How will you push yourself out of your comfort zone?

CHAPTER 6

UNITED KINGDOM:
Musharrat Jabeen Ahmed-Landeryou

Musharrat appears on the screen with short soft blue hair, a black blouse, black over-ear headphones, and giant palm fronds shifting on her virtual background. A British Bangladeshi woman and occupational therapy educator since 2002, Musharrat Jabeen Ahmed-Landeryou was recently promoted in April 2022 to Associate Professor at London South Bank University in England's busy and culturally rich capital.

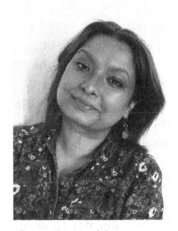

Figure 6.1: Headshot of Musharrat J. Ahmed-Landeryou

Describing London, she starts with "colonialism, the Commonwealth and class that interferes with economics, politics, and has hidden racism in its structures." This leads to inequity and injustice. There's a rich history that seems sophisticated, but underneath it, only a few are privileged while the rest are struggling. She points to all the things tourists come to see and love, but they don't know the truth. The nation's wealth is built on the blood of enslaved people and those colonized by Britain (Anthony, 2021). There are also positive contributions to society from this nation, like the origins of the modern unions we know today began in England. In general, it is a civic-minded society in support of people, whether British or immigrants, yet due to coloniality, racism still runs deep. This statement sums up the proper and polite exterior that contains a brutal legacy of inflicting pain.

Born in Bangladesh, Musharrat moved to Tanzania, England, the United Arab Emirates, and back to England, which made settling in any one place challenging. Her surgeon father had difficulty finding permanent positions, being Muslim and visibly South Asian, so the family moved around for his work. These shifts exposed her to many cultures, languages, and ways of life.

When her family returned to England from the United Arab Emirates, Musharrat shortened her name to Mish, something she had thought about doing for a long time. At university, people had a difficult time with her name. Tired of mispronunciations, she told people to call her Mish. It was much easier, and they caught on quickly. This fostered a sense of belonging in Westernized spaces, so she kept the name until recently.

After watching the *My name is* documentary series about lived experiences with non-Western names, she reclaimed her given name. She attempted this back in 2021 but received little support from peers. In fact, a white co-worker refused and instead made a disparaging comment when Musharrat reintroduced herself using her birth name, requesting peers to use it instead. However, this co-worker recently retired, so when she decided to try again, her colleagues were more supportive and are now respectfully calling her Musharrat.

Her journey to occupational therapy wasn't planned. Before graduating with a degree in physics, she realized her heart wasn't in it. In her final year, she went to the career office and asked for help finding alternatives. The vocational assessment recommended healthcare, and the person in the office helping her suggested she try volunteering. So, after graduation, she started volunteering to find her path, spending time working in day centers. The last place was an adult day center for people with profound learning disabilities and severe physical disabilities. Feeling at ease in this place, she worked five days a week unpaid for a short while until she was offered a full-time job as a low-wage support worker alongside occupational therapy assistants and a lead occupational therapist. The head therapist convinced her to make a career change, encouraging her to study occupational therapy. So, she decided to get a bachelor's degree in occupational therapy, which was very different from her traditional science background.

There are a few paths to becoming an occupational therapist in the UK. There are part-time and full-time undergraduate courses, part-time apprenticeships, or a two-year full-time master's option. Flexible part-time programs allow parents, caregivers, and people who have to work an opportunity to attend the program. A clinical doctorate pathway has been approved as well. These are all ways to get to the same endpoint, allowing for better inclusion in who can become an occupational therapist. In the UK, occupational therapy assistants are not required to gain certification to practice.

I ask Musharrat about her thoughts on the possibility of a doctorate program, as I have strong opinions. In the US, a bachelor's degree is no longer an option for entry. Master's programs are being replaced with doctorate programs as a requirement to enter the profession, thus increasing the barriers to qualification and excluding more people.

In addition, these expensive, high-barrier programs force the profession to be increasingly white, moving from 80 percent at the master's level to 85 percent at the doctoral level, in a country with a 76 percent white population (American Occupational Therapy Association, 2018; US Census Bureau, 2022). We both agree that a clinical doctorate is about status and making money, furthering inequities in occupational therapy.

When Musharrat attended occupational therapy school, only four Black, Asian, and minority ethnic (B.A.M.E.) students were in her program compared to when she was studying physics and diverse representation was the norm. In physics, she studied with international students of varied genders and backgrounds. Moving to occupational therapy, she was learning about care catering to white patients taught by predominantly white women. In the UK, white occupational therapist representation is 10 percent higher than the population representation (The OT Magazine, 2020). In Musharrat's experience, despite living in a culturally diverse society, there was no cultural integration in what she was taught. Disability was a big focus in the program, but not culture. Textbooks used pictures and graphics of primarily white people, reinforcing the message that Musharrat didn't belong. At the time, she didn't speak up about racism and lack of diversity, feeling uncomfortable doing so, and focusing instead on surviving school.

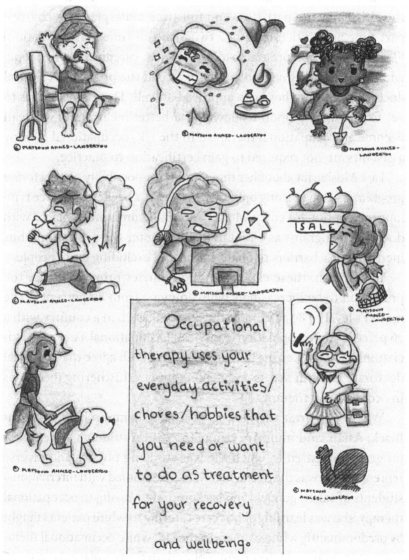

Figure 6.2: Image of diverse representation of occupations, which Musharrat's daughter, Maysoun, drew in response to an all-white appearing representation graphic on the Occupational Therapy Hub website

Finally making a place for herself in a field where she doesn't feel she belongs, Musharrat is focused on challenging the white centering of occupational therapy. After years of not being heard and recognizing that students like her have been unfairly treated, she decided it was time for change. For example, when B.A.M.E. students complain about racism in a clinical placement, they are often pulled out, yet nothing happens to their supervisor. Instead, the placement is maintained for future students to be harmed potentially, and the students who complained have to start over, delaying their completion of the program.

The 2020 murder of George Floyd was traumatic for Black and other people of color around the world, and it became a flashpoint for Black Lives Matter and racial justice movements. Massive global protests demanded justice for Floyd's killing and an end to the systemic racism that continues to harm and take countless Black lives. Yet, despite the calls to action, the profession remained silent. Professional organizations like the Royal College of Occupational Therapists (RCOT) failed to acknowledge that systemic racism within our profession limits access to occupations and appropriate health services that affect health outcomes. As a majority white profession, there is a responsibility to acknowledge the harm done and implement antiracist actions.

Kwaku Agyemang, a British Ghanaian occupational therapist who was a past student of Musharrat's, reached out for guidance. Not having spoken since he was a student almost two years before, he asked for help addressing the lack of concern from the profession. He trusted her out of all the faculty and clinicians he could have approached. Together they decided to protest for active change. Initially, they put a message out on Twitter and received responses from peers from all backgrounds committed to change and working together.

Then, Musharrat and Kwaku wrote an open letter to the RCOT asking for action steps to address racism and inequities in the profession, supported by signatures from 49 peers. Unfortunately, the response they received was impersonal and uncaring, not addressing what they were asking for—accountability and an admission that occupational therapy is institutionally racist. When the leadership of the RCOT changed, they wrote another letter, hoping to be heard this time. Their efforts were organized into BAMEOTUK, a campaign pressure group of racially minoritized staff, students, and educators in the UK, which includes England, Scotland, Wales, and Northern Ireland. The group is growing—originally 20 strong, it now has over 100 regular members. BAMEOTUK is still learning to organize and make an impact as a grassroots, volunteer-run group. Led by Musharrat, they recently held their inaugural virtual symposium, "Equity In Action," with attendees and speakers from around the globe. In addition, they offer regular support groups and educational sessions for racialized students and practitioners.

BAMEOTUK grew out of a need for mutual support for people experiencing racism in the profession, as a way to work together to have their voices heard, and what Musharrat describes as a collaborating space for the potential to co-produce plans and actions for change. This healing space and community validates everyday experiences of racism. Some members didn't realize until they participated in groups that they had faced racism. Their experiences were so normalized that without others sharing that they had gone through the same thing, they were minimizing their own dealings with racism.

Students of color on the verge of failing placements began to reach out to the group. Similar stories were being told. They were failing without any prior notice or warning and finding out near the completion of the internship that they needed better communication skills or weren't socializing with peers, so they weren't going to pass.

Musharrat put on her union hat from her National Health Service days as a union steward and realized that reviewing processes and documentation was key to challenging discriminatory practices. If nothing had been documented about the students' prior mistakes, then something was wrong with the process and system, not the students.

With support from BAMEOTUK members who volunteer their time for mentoring, students have been helped to receive new placements and regain lost confidence. Mentors offer skill-building opportunities, like improving communication, so that over time students will need less help as their confidence and skills grow. This group is helping students meet their competencies and learn how to communicate effectively with supervisors who may not know how to support their communication styles and learning needs.

They also help practicing clinicians with career progression through coaching, mock interviews, and providing resources for getting promotions. So far, they have a 100 percent success rate with promotions for everyone they have worked with. These professionals are qualified for advancements but lack opportunities and support because B.A.M.E. representation is limited in higher positions.

Due to BAMEOTUK's persistence in their activism and demands, the RCOT hired an equality, diversity, and belonging leader and formed a steering group with representatives from B.A.M.E., lesbian, gay, bisexual, transgender, intersex, queer, asexual and other sexually or gender diverse people (LGBTQIA+), and disabled communities.

A year after BAMEOTUK came together, additional affinity groups formed inspired by their leadership and footprint, including LGBTQIA+OTUK and AbleOTUK, representing queer and disabled therapists and students. None of the groups felt represented by the RCOT or the profession. Brought together by their experiences with discrimination in education programs and practice, the three affinity groups work together and pressure the RCOT to support minoritized and marginalized students, practitioners, and service users. Still, there is significant resistance to change and sharing power.

Soon after Kwaku reached out to her, B.A.M.E. allied health students at her university—students she didn't know and had never interacted with—found Musharrat's brown face in the limited pool of faculty of color on the school's website and emailed her. They wanted to know what the university and allied health programs were doing to address systemic racism. So she arranged a meeting with almost 100 B.A.M.E. students. Out of the gathering came requests for faculty involvement and supportive affinity spaces. Working with students in the program, Musharrat formed affinity groups to create an open and safe space for students to access support and talk about issues together with the faculty.

Used to working quietly without much attention, Musharrat has become more publicly vocal on forums like Twitter, which, along with support, attracts negative attention and personal attacks. Yet, as necessary as the work of antiracism and anti-oppression is, building communities of support is mostly arduous unpaid labor that also comes with resistance.

Musharrat (2022) co-wrote a well-received article, "Discussions on co-creating a decolonial approach for an antiracist framework in occupational therapy," in *Occupational Therapy Now*, and is in the process of publishing a textbook on antiracism in occupational therapy, *Antiracist Occupational Therapy: Unsettling the Status Quo* (Ahmed-Landeryou, 2023a). The book is written for the white majority of occupational therapists and therapists of color that are content with the status quo. Chapters are written primarily by authors of color, with an allyship chapter written by white authors calling out to other white professionals to get involved in antiracism work together with peers of color. It examines who is being represented in occupational therapy, how safety and belonging are created, and offers space to challenge and critique education and practice and formulate antiracist actions. Musharrat frames this as creating a re-imagined occupational therapy.

All the work she has described so far is voluntary, outside her paid professional role. In her official work role as an associate professor, Musharrat recently received a year's break from lecturing to work on decolonizing the allied health professions curriculum at her university. During this time, she developed a decolonizing guide to deeply interrogate the curriculum, help people critically reflect on areas, and give them a place to start (Ahmed-Landeryou, 2023b). Students were at the center of her work prioritizing the voices of the most harmed and minoritized.

The process of decolonizing the curriculum for allied health professionals in her university has been challenging, as there is resistance within the department from colleagues. It is as complex as transforming a legacy, especially in a country that claims that racism is not a problem (Office of the United Nations High Commissioner for Human Rights, 2021). Nevertheless, in this short time, she has managed to arrange for students working on the decolonizing project to be paid for their work, encouraged the faculty to incorporate more global perspectives in the programs by assigning international articles, and built in an option for students to choose an alternative assessment method to make assessments more accessible. An example of this is submitting an audio recording of an essay instead of writing, though accessible alternatives are continuously developing.

Over the last two years, Musharrat has been more immersed in the occupational therapy community in higher education, as she is trying to expand decolonizing the curriculum within the UK. She started a WhatsApp group for this, with shared resources, a space to communicate updates and offer support for this challenging work, and an opportunity to learn from mistakes together. It's a community consisting of mainly white peers. The positive updates in other programs bring her some hope for the profession.

A late-blooming activist, she is compelled to create and be involved in as many communities as possible to spotlight racism and what antiracism actions look like. It wasn't safe, and there weren't enough people willing to speak up publicly before, but doors have since opened. In addition, her own experiences with racism allow her to support others who have experienced similar harm.

Musharrat insists that occupational therapy is political, and activist roles are necessary. For those who disagree, she recommends reading the 2008 text, *A Political Practice of Occupational Therapy* (Pollard *et al.*, 2008). Activism is not about destroying but enhancing a sense of belonging in the profession, with equitable global representation, rather than promoting white-centric occupational therapy worldwide. Speaking with Global South occupational therapists about their challenges, she recognizes that they were taught a monocultural, Western occupational therapy. They have to translate it to make it work with the people in their communities.

Antiracism and anti-discrimination must be embedded in occupational therapy professional practice and education. By not doing this, we are condoning the racism that the profession perpetuates. Musharrat's advice to readers is to understand the history of colonialism, antiracism movements, health disparities, and inequity in relation to occupational therapy before trying to change anything. She recommends several resources, including "Decolonising occupation:

Causing social change to help our ancestors rest and our descendants thrive" by Isla Emery-Whittington and Ben Te Maro (2018), "Occupational consciousness" and further work by Professor Elelwani Ramugondo (2015), the BAMEOTUK YouTube channel, the *South Asian OT Experience* podcast, the *OT & Chill* podcast, DisruptOT recordings, and the first edition of *Occupational Therapy Without Borders* (Kronenberg *et al.*, 2005).

As occupational therapists, we are concerned with service users thriving, but it should be a part of our training to care for each other as well. Musharrat is still trying to find that sense of belonging in the profession. However, she has felt a stronger sense of belonging for the first time in 30 years after connecting with the international occupational therapy community. She is dedicated to unlearning the Eurocentric ways she was taught in her formal education and enhancing this with new learnings on global decoloniality.

SUGGESTED NEXT STEPS

Reflection: What does an antiracist approach to occupational therapy look like in your region?

Action: What steps will you take to deliver an antiracist practice?

References

Ahmed-Landeryou, M., Emery-Whittington, I., Ivlev, S.R., & Elder, R. (2022). "Discussions on co-creating a decolonial approach for an antiracist framework in occupational therapy." *Occupational Therapy Now*, 25: 14–17.

Ahmed-Landeryou, M. (2023a). *Antiracist Occupational Therapy: Unsettling the Status Quo.* London and Philadelphia, PA: Jessica Kingsley Publishers.

Ahmed-Landeryou, M. (2023b). "Developing an evidence-Informed decolonising curriculum wheel – A reflective piece." *Equity in Education & Society*, 0(0), https://doi.org/10.1177/27526461231154014.

American Occupational Therapy Association. (2018). *Academic Programs Annual Data Report: Academic Year 2017–2018.* www.aota.org/~/media/Corporate/Files/EducationCareers/Educators/2017-2018-Annual-Data-Report.pdf.

Anthony, A. (2021). "Blood Legacy by Alex Renton review—family fortunes built on brutality." *The Guardian.* www.theguardian.com/books/2021/may/23/blood-legacy-by-alex-renton-review-family-fortunes-built-on-brutality.

Emery-Whittington, I. & Te Maro, B. (2018). "Decolonising occupation: Causing social change to help our ancestors rest and our descendants thrive." *New Zealand Journal of Occupational Therapy*, 65(1): 12–19.

Kronenberg, F., Algado, S.S., & Pollard, N. (2005). *Occupational Therapy Without Borders*. Edinburgh: Churchill Livingstone.

Office of the United Nations High Commissioner for Human Rights. (2021). *UN Experts Condemn UK Commission on Race and Ethnic Disparities Report*. www.ohchr.org/en/press-releases/2021/04/un-experts-condemn-uk-commission-race-and-ethnic-disparities-report.

Pollard, N., Sakellariou, D., & Kronenberg, F. (2008). *A Political Practice of Occupational Therapy*. Edinburgh: Churchill Livingstone.

Ramugondo, E.L. (2015). "Occupational consciousness." *Journal of Occupational Science*, 22(4): 488–501.

The OT Magazine. (2020). "Changing the face of OT." https://ot-magazine.co.uk/changing-the-face-of-ot.

US Census Bureau QuickFacts: United States. (2022). www.census.gov/quickfacts/fact/table/US/PST045222.

CHAPTER 7

AOTEAROA NEW ZEALAND: Isla Te Ara o Rehua Emery-Whittington

It's hard not to feel at ease when meeting with Isla. Her pleasant virtual background, gently flowing waves and a single palm tree shifting in the breeze match her thoughtful words and flow. Isla Te Ara o Rehua Emery-Whittington introduces herself by sharing landmarks, "Ko Tainui te waka, Ko Kakepuku te maunga, Ko Waipa te awa, Ko Ngāti Maniapoto te iwi, Tēnā koutou, tēnā tātou katoa. [Tainui is my canoe. My mountain is Kakepuku. My river is called Waipa. My people are of Maniapoto and our home space is called Te Kōpua. Greetings to us all.]"

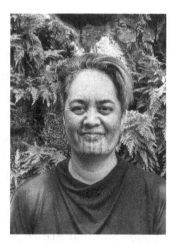

Figure 7.1: Isla standing in front of lithophytes and greenery near her home

She has short, straight, two-toned hair, the black brushed back with a blonde fringe laying off to one side in front, and *moko kauwae*, the traditional chin tattoo for Māori women, visible from her bottom lip down her chin.

A Māori occupational therapist of over 25 years, she is indigenous to Tāmaki Makaurau, Aotearoa (Auckland, New Zealand), and lives there with her husband and three children. Tāmaki Makaurau, the Māori name for Auckland, is located between two harbors, the west and east coast separated by only three kilometers, surrounded by water. The larger city of Auckland is also known as the Polynesian capital of the world. Along with Māori, there are Samoan, Tongan, Cook Islanders, Niuean, Tokelau, Tuvalu, and Fijian peoples, numbering over a quarter million (Auckland Council, n.d.).

Isla grew up in south Auckland within the northern tribal boundaries of Tainui. Her father worked at a national boarding school and institution for low-vision and partially sighted children, and the family lived on-site. Residential institutions were common then, and she and her sister were the only sighted children at the school. In a unique and early introduction to a health and education setting, Isla was also exposed to various therapists and rehabilitation professionals.

Māori have a rich oral history and tradition of storytelling. Valuing and keeping to traditional ways, Isla is a remarkable and engaging storyteller. From memory, she tells me about colonial history, including the early arrival of Europeans in the late 1700s, the 1835 Declaration of Independence, and the 1840 treaty called Te Tiriti o Waitangi. These histories are relevant to life and her work today.

In 1835, the Declaration of Independence was signed by *hapū* (subtribes) chiefs throughout the country as, at that time, Māori politics were *hapū* based, not tribal as they are today. The Declaration affirmed continued *hapū* sovereignty over the islands and made international trade easier. In 1840, a treaty was signed with Britain, which wanted to send more people. The treaty meant ongoing sovereignty of *hapū* and that British arrivals would be ruled under British laws. In return, Māori would also have the same rights as British subjects, and, if chiefs ever sold land, a cultural impossibility, the Crown would offer a fair price. Within months, the treaty was dishonored by the British, who organized a settler government primarily to extract land and were ready for war against Māori who would not sell.

Before the treaty, Māori were in good health, successfully trading and growing crops to feed new settlers. One tribe had its own bank and international trading links. When the treaty was signed, there were over 200,000 Māori and 2000 white people. This is a stark difference from Māori life today, with current demographics of 70 percent white and 17.4 percent Māori (Statistics New Zealand Tatauranga Aotearoa, 2018; Statistics New Zealand Tatauranga Aotearoa, 2022) and systemic racism and the impacts of colonization resulting in disproportionately high levels of poverty and poor health (Hobbs *et al.*, 2019).

Te Tiriti is an amazing social justice document that allowed white settlers to govern themselves and live as they were used to while affirming the continuation of Māori sovereignty and way of life. Te Tiriti o Waitangi is the internationally recognized legal text, while The Treaty of Waitangi, the English version, is not. Despite the English version being an inaccurate illegal translation of Te Tiriti, this is the version preferred by settler governments. Most New Zealanders, including occupational therapists, receive minimal Tiriti education in school.

Isla teaches in a postgraduate mental health and addiction program and is a Tiriti, decolonization, and antiracism trainer. She has worked with various health organizations, supporting their education and regulatory requirements. Her approach to teaching people about Māori and Māori health begins with unlearning stereotypes about Māori and learning about colonization, racism, and Te Tiriti. This is necessary learning for anyone living in the country, but "like many settler colonial states, citizens do not know local history, and this is by design," she illuminates.

When Isla was 14, her cousin, who was 9, sustained a traumatic head injury, and fearing the worst, the family was told to say goodbye. However, he survived surgery and recovered in a rehabilitation facility for some years. It was a relief to have him home, but the house had to undergo modifications that an occupational therapist oversaw. When Isla asked her cousin who his favorite therapist was, he said it was the occupational therapist because she helped him do what he wanted to do.

Isla had a close and large family, and a Christmas tradition included opening presents together. One Christmas day, Isla's grandfather pointed to each of the older *mokopuna* (grandchildren) and told them what he thought they would be when they grew up.

He based his guesses and guidance on what he observed of each child's character. Isla was told she would be a nurse. He wasn't far off.

In time, Isla applied to physical and occupational therapy programs and was accepted to both. She laughs, remembering that she chose the occupational therapy program because they sent their acceptance letter first. Isla studied at the Auckland Institute of Technology, which later became the Auckland University of Technology, situated on the North Shore. In this predominantly white area, white settlers, even recent ones, tend to congregate, as reflected in continued overrepresentation on campus.

In contrast, few Māori choose to study occupational therapy. Isla recalls how some of her peers repeatedly and publicly asked how she managed to get onto the program. It was her first time in a predominantly white space, so that kind of open racism was stunning and confusing. These would be future occupational therapists. Looking back, Isla can see they didn't think she belonged and that she was taking the place of a white student who was, in their minds, more deserving. Isla remembers no faculty intervening when students expressed racist ideas, but she did feel supported by the then head of school, Gail Whiteford, an Australian woman.

As a new graduate, Isla was hired for six hours a week to support Māori student retention and recruitment. Isla's office was converted from the janitor's closet and was situated by the toilets. As with other professions, when Māori identify as Māori, it attracts pigeonholing and peculiar requests by non-Māori that can sometimes create culturally unsafe and spiritually compromising situations. For instance, as a student she would open conferences using Māori customs, more appropriate for a seasoned Māori occupational therapist. So in 2002, when her husband's company secured contracts in Birmingham, UK, Isla was ready to move. The much-needed change from being hyper-visible and *the* token Māori occupational therapist allowed Isla to have some cultural anonymity and grow as an occupational therapist.

In almost 55 years of occupational therapy in Aotearoa New Zealand, Isla was one of the first ten Māori occupational therapists. Currently, there are nearly 300 Māori occupational therapists in

Aotearoa. Māori are 17.4 percent of the population but make up 6 percent of occupational therapists (Statistics New Zealand Tatauranga Aotearoa, 2022). Unfortunately, this data on students is nearly impossible to obtain, creating an even greater obstacle toward equitable representation.

In 2004, Isla was contacted by new graduate Māori practitioners and asked to provide supervision. Instead, she suggested a peer supervision arrangement as the collective aspect of supervision was more in keeping with *tikanga Māori*—Māori customary practices. This collective has come to be known as The Māori Occupational Therapy Network and aims to meet monthly in a safe space to support and develop practitioners as Māori in the profession. Māori protocols are prioritized and practiced. A regular feature is processing and healing from racist experiences during training and practice. Depending on who heads the occupational therapy program, students experience a variable degree of access to the Network, which actively supports and mentors Māori students, including offering fieldwork placements. Most students who connect to the Network remain active members following graduation.

Numbers fluctuate, and Isla estimates that over 120 Māori occupational therapists and students have been part of the Network. People come for different reasons; some have specific goals, some just want to be together, some ask for help with issues, and some see the Network as a source of "free" cultural advisors. This aspect has become problematic, so now the Network seeks an understanding of intentions and supports people to grasp the shape of their contribution.

For Māori, land is central to identity, providing an economic, political, and spiritual base. Greetings often start with naming landmarks like the mountain and river. "The land tells you who you are," Isla explains. "These are our grandparents. These are who fed, housed, and sheltered our ancestors—some still do. The mountains, rivers, seas looked after us for centuries, and they know who you are even if you don't." She summarizes, "If coming to a Māori OT Network meeting is the most Māori thing you do, there's a need to also go home and find out who you are."

A growing frustration, many professionals make excuses for not taking action in antiracism and decolonization work. Isla contrasts how the Network moves forward while so many others remain tied to the status quo, "Feeling powerless to act is a theme I hear all too often in occupational therapy. This is exactly what colonialism and its newer form, neoliberalism, want us to think and feel. They [Māori Occupational Therapy Network] never feel powerless to act, probably because we gather and to gather is its own medicine. We look after one another, celebrate the wins, inevitably feel angry and then act. But we've continued to do as we choose. It is our own power, our mana, that no one can take away."

Throughout her career, Isla has switched between Māori ways of being, doing, and speaking with Māori service users in Māori Health Services, and white ways in mainstream healthcare. Like many Māori occupational therapists, she has learned Māori occupational therapies outside and despite mainstream training and practice that cater to settlers.

Done well, occupational therapy services for Māori and non-Māori require the practitioner to offer different ways of being with people. Conversely, establishing relationships is integral to being in good relations with everyone and everything. This is reflected in bringing respectful formality initially when meeting a person and *whānau* (family group). When Isla worked for a tribal health service, morning *karakia* (prayers or invocations) connected staff to gods, ancestors, purpose, and each other when starting each day. This was followed by a short welcome of words and a song that helped staff focus their good intentions and bestow safety. To end, thanks were offered to whoever had led the gathering that day. The ritual is brief—about 15 minutes—and is standard practice in Māori health settings.

I ask how this might look in a hospital. "You get good and fast at it," she assures me. Depending on the space, Māori practitioners greet Māori cheerfully, "Kia ora!" It is not possible to complete a full welcome, but it is possible to greet everyone supporting that person and bring good energy to the space. The practitioner first introduces themselves by sharing where they are from, and the *whānau* will do the same. By this stage, a connection or commonality is usually established—that is, how they may know each other, who they might know in common, and how they might be related to each other (a common ancestor). "Our words guide us in how to be with each other. For instance, *whānau* means family group as well as to give birth. *Whanaunga* means a cousin/relation, and *whanaungatanga* means to create family and connection." Creating connections in healthcare, *whakawhanaungatanga*, is about valuing being in relation with while knowing who you are. Isla explains, "It's like the fern knowing the pine and the fungi as neighbors and each understanding how they exist in relation to each other." Subsequently, it is common for Māori practitioners to know of familial and/or community relationships to staff and clients because knowing where they are from is highly valued and practiced. This is seen as a "conflict" in some western-based healthcare services.

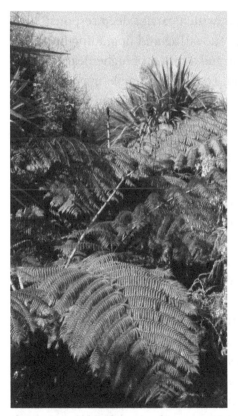

Figure 7.2: Local plants growing near Isla's home

At one tribal health service, Isla shares that the mental health initial assessment begins with the entire service team—occupational therapist, psychologist, nurse, social worker, family advocate, and receptionist—meeting with the person seeking care and their *whānau*. Overall, assessment and treatment take less time, despite a longer welcome than in mainstream settings, because time is spent growing relationships and understanding concerns from *whānau* perspectives. This allows for time to build trust and learn their stories. Standard mental health assessments are still offered, but they are only a piece of the relationship, not the full story. Because colonization is understood as a constant force and a social determinant of health, the biopsychosocial model is flipped and becomes the cultural-social-psycho-bio model. Care options are left open and include Western and tribal healing choices.

Isla is a trustee of her *hapū*, which carries deep responsibility. The *hapū* is in the process of renovating and upgrading buildings and planning for a health clinic and a center of higher learning that includes language revitalization. The *hapū* is completing research for this monumental project which will include a closed waste system that entails catching rainwater, purifying it for drinking, growing food and plant medicine, and rehabilitating land and river.

I ask Isla if this vision includes an occupational therapy program. The answer is complicated. "The *hapū* will partner with the best Indigenous university that fits our needs. In terms of occupational therapy, though, our registration body is currently researching the possibility of an Indigenous occupational therapy program with one of the three Māori universities." The Māori Occupational Therapy Network is not formally included in the research and set-up, however. Isla explains that when looking for Māori occupational therapy expertise, Māori occupational therapists can be overlooked for Māori who might have expertise in teaching non-Māori about Māori culture and traditions. These are two very different functions but are often seen as the same by non-Māori.

There is an assumption from the predominantly white leaders that Māori occupational therapists are very colonized and Westernized, unconnected to their roots, without language and traditions. "Yet, critical thinking, *tikanga*-led practitioner numbers are increasing," and are active members of the Network and have decades of combined knowledge of how to work well with their own in decolonizing ways. Another assumption is that non-Māori are equipped to assess how Māori one is or is not. Conversely, Māori occupational therapists walk in both worlds, code-switching seamlessly, because they are Māori who chose to study occupational therapy. Exasperated, after a long pause, Isla explains, "Too much of my time in occupational therapy spaces has been taken up teaching white people how to 'be with' and engage us without harming us."

Isla acknowledges that there's a difference in education and critical examination between a Māori occupational therapist and an occupational therapist who happens to be Māori. Similarly, there is a difference between a Māori researcher and a *Kaupapa Māori* researcher. *Kaupapa Māori* research insists on transformational practice and that "Māori are benefiting during and as an outcome of the study." Isla clarifies that it is done by, with, and for Māori and informed by *tikanga* Māori.

For some years, Isla has prepared and shared decolonization, *Kaupapa Māori* theory, and studies with the Network. She then realized that the development of ideas taking place among the members of the Network needed to be formalized. However, there was no existing infrastructure in occupational therapy education that could hold Māori knowledges. A space would need to be carved out. So, Isla approached a well-known and well-regarded *Kaupapa Maori* researcher who saw the potential of decolonizing everyday occupations to fit the Māori context. The Network provides social and spiritual guidance for the study, as do some essential international Indigenous and critical colleagues. A usual practice in *Kaupapa Māori* research is to gather a *kaitiaki* (guardian) group, and for Isla's study, that includes a Māori occupational therapist, a tribal representative, a family representative, and a *Pākeha* (non-Māori of European descent) occupational therapist scholar whom she trusts. Ethics approval is also sought from *whānau* and *hapū*. It is considered more important because "colonization via research has a long history with Indigenous peoples," and Western ethics address different concerns.

Isla describes her study as being informed by both occupational science and occupational therapy because it centers a Māori understanding of human doing, and the *Kaupapa Māori* theory and practice model is aimed at supporting practitioners. Given the presence of unmitigated racism in occupational therapy and occupational science and the lack of theorizing about it, Isla realized that the developing theory and practice model needs antiracism designed within it. She explains that the developing theory concerns *mahi*, not occupation alone. "*Mahi* is a physical and tangible manifestation of what has existed in the spiritual realm and what we humans now do, and who we are. *Mahi* expands on and includes occupation and is what gods, creatures, and then humans do, in that order. Beyond activities, *mahi* is about contributing to all creation, serving others, and how good relations are expressed." Therefore, she reveals, *mahi* is politically, socially, geographically, and spiritually contextual.

I ask Isla what she loves about her study, and her immediate response is, "I love figuring out whiteness." She references Linda Tuhiwai Smith's 2012 book *Decolonizing Methodologies: Research and Indigenous Peoples*, discussing *Kaupapa Māori* research's role in turning the lens from "us and back onto whiteness," the opposite of anthropologists (or occupational scientists) who study the "other." Isla's study examines how oppression is naturalized via everyday occupation. From a *Kaupapa Māori mahi* lens, she can see that racism has become ordinary in everyday life. Her analysis helps her family understand things happening around them and then bring *hapū* practices, stories, knowledge, and objects back into everyday life. This is the greater meaning of her studies and work.

The biggest misconception about occupational therapy in New Zealand is that it is a bicultural practice setting. "We're a long way from that, and I am concerned about the colonial messaging that has gone global about how great our race relations are here. Who benefits from this story or 'look'? Who needs this story to be true? Just scratch the surface, and the truth will be revealed."

I ask Isla if she feels as if she belongs in the profession. "I know I don't. Just turning up—just existing—is challenging for some, and this is before I open my mouth. If being Māori is such a challenge, then occupational therapy really needs to have a reckoning with itself...it needs a rebuild." She wants us to "have a moment of truth" and admit to all levels of racism ingrained in the profession. "You can't heal without truth," she insists. "It is hard, but it is past time to carve out a space and make it easier for Māori, Indigenous peoples, the global majority who want to practice and for our many communities that require this profession's support."

While discussing her hopes for occupational therapy, a tabby cat's tail cuts across the screen, breaking through the virtual illusion of her sitting beside calm waters. She wants non-Māori leaders to "get out of the way. The Māori Occupational Therapy Network knows what we need to do and what our community needs of us." The focus must shift to ensuring that Māori experience an equitable occupational therapy education and service and have as many treatment options as everyone else. The priority has for too long been about catching non-Māori up, educating them before they harm, and trying to heal what harm has happened while preventing more.

This opens past wounds. Isla looks down, asking her cat Peow-Peow not to drool on her while petting him. It's a tiny moment of levity, and we continue a tough conversation. "I've got way more hope in the global occupational therapy community because they haven't been taught to hate Māori yet," she says as we both awkwardly laugh, the reality being too intense to sit quietly with. "I have way more hope because of DisruptOT, more hope than I've ever had." She wants more community building, a community that shares, without capitalism or competition, and enjoys being together. Decolonization can happen more realistically together as a global community.

Colonization has touched all of us, considering the roots of occupational therapy and the same white-centered ways of practice spread across the globe, with Western textbooks, theories, practices, and the World Federation of Occupational Therapists sanctioning rote Western program standards worldwide.

Isla believes that if Te Tiriti o Waitangi was understood and honored, recognition and acceptance that everyone does things differently, for an understandable reason, would be the standard. Recognizing the sovereignty of each *hapū* means there is no need to impose one way over another. Each is allowed to be and exist, as *hapū* did for centuries prior to colonization. She wants this cultivation of relationships from non-Māori, as the Tiriti was set up to do, "We can assume that people have tried things and figured out what works and what doesn't. We won't know why everyone does what they do, but we can assume people are doing the best with what they have."

SUGGESTED NEXT STEPS

Reflection: What do you know about the Indigenous peoples of the lands you are living, teaching, or working in? Think about what you know and have heard and examine this. For example, who shared this information (from whose perspective), and who benefits from how the stories are told?

Action: Take time to identify your roots, history, and surrounding landmarks. What is the significance of these to you as a person and professional?

References

Auckland Council. (n.d.). *Tāmaki Makaurau Moananui-ā-Kiwa*. Pacific Auckland. www.aucklandcouncil.govt.nz/plans-projects-policies-reports-bylaws/our-plans-strategies/auckland-plan/about-the-auckland-plan/Pages/pacific-auckland.aspx.

Hobbs, M., Ahuriri-Driscoll, A., Marek, L., Campbell, M., Tomintz, M., & Kingham, S. (2019). "Reducing health inequity for Māori people in New Zealand." *The Lancet*, 394(10209), 1613–1614, https://doi.org/10.1016/s0140-6736(19)30044-3.

Smith, L.T. (2012). *Decolonizing Methodologies: Research and Indigenous Peoples* (second edition). London and New York, NY: Zed Books.

Statistics New Zealand Tatauranga Aotearoa (2018). *2018 Census place summaries*. www.stats.govt.nz/tools/2018-census-place-summaries/new-zealand.

Statistics New Zealand Tatauranga Aotearoa (2022). Māori population estimates: At 30 June 2022. www.stats.govt.nz/information-releases/maori-population-estimates-at-30-june-2022.

CHAPTER 8

UNITED STATES: Adam Cisroe Pearson

Adam Cisroe Pearson lives in St. Louis, Missouri, in the Midwest of the United States (US). Living in what's considered the Bible Belt, a Black, progressive housing advocate like him might seem out of place. He is married with a seven-year-old daughter and a three-year-old son. Religion is an important part of his identity. An Episcopalian Christian, at times he has been agnostic, questioning his beliefs while recognizing there is a creator.

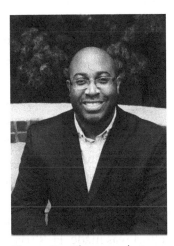

Figure 8.1: Close-up photo of Adam sitting outside

Working in community mental health in homeless services as the Chief Operating Officer of Peter & Paul Community Services, he oversees housing, shelter programs, and around 80 staff members. The organization's mission, "we walk with people facing homelessness on their journey to lifelong stability," alludes to their scope of services.

The nature of this work requires long hours, working nights and weekends when problems arise. Fortunately, Adam enjoys solving the program's complex dilemmas, which require him to be creative and available in dire situations. For instance, recently, a packed shelter was flooded, and he had to work to find alternative accommodations for everyone until the damage was remediated.

He was drawn to homeless services in 2010 as a graduate occupational therapy student in downtown St. Louis. The city was evicting residents of "Hopeville," a community of unhoused people living in an abandoned railway tunnel under Tucker Boulevard. Plans to rebuild the road and seal the tunnel would leave them without shelter. In a controversial move, a major shelter provider staged a protest by moving people into the tunnel. This created a media frenzy, now covering the eviction of about 100 people, including children and families. The city and another homeless services organization had to provide case management and short-term housing to get people out of the tunnel.

Adam read about it in the paper and decided to go down to the tunnel on eviction day and see the situation for himself. Genuinely curious and concerned, he spoke with people and asked questions. That was the day he knew he wanted to work in homeless services, navigating and solving what he calls a "massive puzzle" of political complications with people trapped in the middle. Adam estimates that St. Louis has five times as many empty homes sitting around as individuals who need housing. He is fascinated by the challenge of solving the disconnect and getting people who often have mental illness and substance use issues the support they need. As he sees it, people could be placed in housing in less than a year if an honest effort was made. He's trying to make this effort now.

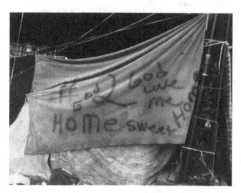

Figure 8.2: Tent structure at the Tucker Tunnel

Adam thought he wanted to be a doctor. Then, during his junior year as a premed major, he began to shadow doctors and was discouraged by the paperwork involved in their day. He set off to explore other options based on his studies and considered allied health professions. Excited by the idea of working with people to help them reach small goals rather than big ones, he decided to pursue occupational therapy.

Occupational therapy school prepared him for the basic components of clinical work. But, he had to learn about public affairs, finance, accounting, tax credits, and fundraising—the art of convincing a politician they should fund your program. This is something he has grown to excel in. The structure of local politics impacts the people and communities we work with, yet none of this is taught in occupational therapy programs. He credits community advocates he has worked with and on-the-job training for helping him pick up these essential skills.

Adam grew up in Normandy, about a mile and a half away from Ferguson, Missouri, where Michael Brown, an unarmed Black teenager, was shot and killed by a police officer in 2014, fueling protests around the country. The white officer who shot him was never charged. Though he was raised in a middle-class neighborhood, Adam spent much time in lower-income communities with food insecurity and poor housing stability. Here in north St. Louis, his friends and their families experienced issues similar to the homeless and newly unhoused people he works with, such as not having enough money to meet basic needs for food and housing. These intimate experiences made it easier to understand and talk to people in the shelters—skills that can't be taught in school. Building connection and trust have been far more critical to his work than any book or school learning.

After graduating, he became a community practice clinician, a role that included working in a drop-in day shelter. There, he developed supportive programs and completed needs assessments and evaluations. Taking up a management position for the first time, Adam went to work for Peter & Paul Community Services (PPCS) to design a fully accessible supportive housing facility from an abandoned elementary school, including building a large team to run housing and clinical support.

He left for a stint in the political sector, but missing working directly with people impacted by the things he was advocating for, he applied for a leadership role as Chief Operating Officer with PPCS. Currently, he is the only occupational therapist in the organization. I was stunned, assuming there was an occupational therapy department this whole time. However, they recently put occupational therapy in their budget, and Adam plans to help grow that team. Many other services support clients, such as counselors, nurses, life skills specialists, and social workers.

Also, a faculty member, Adam likes to teach about "real-life shit" because a sole focus on activities of daily living is not sufficient or appropriate for this population. If someone doesn't have access to a safe place to sleep or food to eat, how much will they care about an occupational therapy session addressing activities of daily living?

Examples of interventions he's facilitated and subsequently taught students about include engaging with a person actively using crack cocaine, as in holding a crack pipe and crack in their hands while an occupational therapist is working with them; working with a sex worker on safety and access to contraception; prioritizing access to sustenance after walking into a client's home and finding out their baby has not been fed for a day. School and internships did not prepare him for these situations, and in reality, these are situations where students and clinicians are often afraid or offended. Yet, these are real-life situations with no threat to the therapist. We should be prepared to navigate these situations with respect and knowledge on how to best support the people involved. Though a case study or simulation can introduce students to these challenging situations, hands-on learning opportunities are the only way to navigate them.

Adam often lectures to students and practitioners about harm reduction, which is a method of reducing harm where possible with drug use while respecting the rights of people who use drugs. Another real-life example he gives is budgeting for drugs, an instrumental activity of daily living, similar to budgeting for food. Improper budgeting will negatively affect their ability to pay rent. This makes some students uncomfortable, but it is occupational therapy in the real world. Even occupations we are unfamiliar or uncomfortable with fall within our scope of practice and job responsibility when the people we work with prioritize them. Adam thrives with these challenging conversations, seeing a potential shift in biases and worldviews as the payoff.

He's planning to expand the occupational therapy department at PPCS to offer students more exposure to working in this sector and help that discomfort to turn into understanding and care—this is a way to help the next generation of therapists be unafraid to address real issues.

The basic definition of occupational therapy he learned in school is what he uses when explaining what he does with people: "engaging in the activities that give you and your life meaning" with the addition of "the activities that you absolutely need to do in order for you to get more stable." Regarding occupations considered illicit, he frames his work to support making them safer.

Some of the biggest challenges he experiences in his line of work at PPCS are finances, fundraising, and fragmentation of municipalities and services. Another issue is apathy, housed neighbors voting down initiatives to build housing and supportive services. It's common for people to call the police on unhoused people, not because they are concerned about safety or health but because they don't want these people near their homes.

Sitting on a white chair with the door closed, Adam, wearing a black t-shirt with black half-rimmed glasses, pauses to check outside the door. He warns me that his son, Phin, might join our talk.

A crying three-year-old with big brown eyes and a buzz cut enters the room, going silent as he sits on his dad's lap, fresh tears falling down his face.

Adam wasn't taught how to connect with people with power and money, noting, "they speak a different language to us." He calls much of what he does "acting," having to connect with hugely wealthy people who are out of touch with what Adam understands and the things people at PPCS experience daily. It is a critical skill to fund his work that he has had to pick up on his own.

With his son on his lap, Adam tells me how dedicated PPCS's staff are and how much they care about clients and their work. In their most challenging times, the clients trust the team. His work is rewarding and complicated, and at times messy. But it's never boring, and when someone finds a home or reconnects with family, he gets to share in their joy and remind himself that the hard work is worth it.

It wasn't until he traveled outside St. Louis that he realized how racist the city is. It is a racially segregated region resembling a "white people sandwich" in the center and Black and other communities of color above and below these sections. St. Louis happens to be one of the most segregated cities in the US. Yet, it was only a few years ago that this became an issue that politicians chose to discuss.

Racial segregation involves income and housing. Unhoused people are likely to be from one of the two bands where most Black St. Louisans live. A former industrial town, the white middle class moved out of the city into the suburbs in what is known as "white flight," happening around major US cities after racial desegregation. Middle-class white families escaped increasingly racially diverse cities, moving to exclusive and growing white suburbs with support from the federal government. Eventually, as Black people were allowed to move into the suburban areas, white families moved back to the city into more economically prosperous neighborhoods, and some ventured further out of the suburbs into more homogenous and wealthy areas outside the metropolitan area.

With significant investments from the city into the midtown corridor of St. Louis to get more affluent people to move in, many of these white suburban residents moved back to the city, filling up the middle region to occupy the new luxury housing built to draw them in. This new type of housing is cost prohibitive to most Black families in the area. Residential racial segregation resulting from redlining is a fundamental cause of racial disparities in health and wealth within the US (Nardone *et al.*, 2020). Redlining was the discriminatory practice of denying mortgages to Black and Indigenous Americans and immigrants while subsidizing the building of white neighborhoods, in which Black people were not allowed to purchase homes. To this day, there are consequences in these predominantly Black and Brown neighborhoods that have not changed in over 50 years after housing discrimination was banned. Historical redlining in the US explains how white families gained generational wealth while Black families were kept from it and are impacted presently.

Traditionally Black neighborhoods are now becoming gentrified, the process of current residents being replaced by wealthy ones moving in, including the area where Adam and his family live. Gentrification, historical redlining, and present-day segregation are a national phenomenon. I live in San Francisco, and studies have shown that not only does historical redlining result in similar present-day racial and income segregation, but health outcomes are worse in neighborhoods predominantly occupied by people of color (Nardone *et al.*, 2020).

In the past, Adam has spent time in religious, conservative, predominantly white regions, connecting with people. Acknowledging valid concern for his safety, he would like to take a year off, move to one of these towns, and talk to all white congregations about racism and their views on race and politics. He thinks it would be energizing yet knows it's terrifying. He grew up in the church, is familiar with church-going ways, and believes he might get through to people, and help them see the humanity in people who don't look like them.

Having worked in three regions of the country with different demographics and political and religious leanings, Adam has had three very different experiences. Though St. Louis is segregated, he finds it more progressive. The Texas Panhandle was hyper-conservative, but he found that people were very nice to him, with the exception of a few overtly racist experiences, such as patients telling him they didn't like Black people and asking to work with someone else because they didn't want a Black therapist. In Springfield, Missouri, as a college student, he experienced open, blatant racism from college students and strangers in the community. Crediting his experience in St. Louis with making him street smart, he believes he can connect with people in a way that isn't intimidating and can break through some of their biases about Black men. Still, he is aware of the boundaries of where he can't visit because those areas were historically unsafe for Black people and still are.

Spending some time as a traveling occupational therapist in "deep red Texas," a region that is predominantly white and votes consistently for conservative leaders and policies that contribute to racial inequity, he's connected with many people and learned about their political views. He learned that a lack of experience with people from different backgrounds heavily influences their political views.

He recalls an incident at work while a college student in Springfield, a predominantly white town. A full-time manager at a residence at the time, he was giving an orientation tour and noticed a white woman moving into the facility looking at him suspiciously. During dinner, she pulled him aside and asked him if he was the janitor. He told her he was the manager, and with a severe tone, she asked, "So, they let coloreds work in management down here?" She had never seen a Black person work in management. Where she was from, it was more common for Black people to work in service roles where they didn't have opportunities to move up.

Despite the segregation and racism in St. Louis, there are plentiful parks and a vibrant international food scene. Adam hopes to visit all of the parks and playgrounds in the city before the year ends. Every neighborhood has at least one park, and they are well funded and maintained, even in low-income areas. This is surprising because most neighborhood parks are funded based on the local property taxes, leaving poor neighborhoods neglected with dilapidated and unsafe recreation spaces. Adam relishes taking his children all over the city to play and meet children from different communities.

I finally catch a smile as Phin plays with his dad's hands.

Less than 1 percent of occupational therapists in the US are Black men. Adam firmly believes the profession does not represent him, his culture, or even the people he works with. With the educational curriculum focused on an idyllic version of occupation, he thinks it will take at least a decade or two of active work on disrupting curriculum to address the real issues people face. He works with people who don't have health insurance or a place to be discharged to after hospitalization where they can continue with recommended occupational therapy plans. The US occupational therapy model—treatment, assessment, and billing—assumes that everyone has insurance and understands the treatment and assessments used.

Spending so much of his time and energy on work, Adam would like to connect more with Black leaders. A small group of Black faculty at his university discuss issues that impact them. Groups like Black-male Registered Occupational Therapy Healthcare-professionals Assistants & Students (BROTHAS) exist to foster belonging, show-case various specialties, grow leadership potential, and amplify representation.

I bluntly ask if he feels as if he belongs in the profession, and he pauses to think about it. He's never been asked this. He points out his privilege as a non-disabled, cisgender man. Being Black knocks that privilege down some. Overall, he's felt welcome, which he credits to his leadership and soft skills in drawing people in. Some Black male occupational therapists he's known were pushed out of the profes-sion, about seven of them. Not everyone has had the success he has. He believes that more Black men in the profession will normalize and acclimate people to working with them, be less intimidated and threatened, and be more likely to notice the value they add to the team.

Like the rest of the world, professionals have biases, but as the profession leans heavily toward white women, views are even more harmful (Steed, 2014). Opportunities to work with more Black men might shift people's experience of working with them, making it a less hostile environment to work in. I recall a story shared by a Black occupational therapist business owner who had had the police called on him frequently while at his established place of work, even when wearing a white lab coat. It happened so often that he'd grown to expect it.

Occupational therapy is political and should be more political. Politics can keep people from engaging in daily activities, so Adam believes we should be more politically aware. As the shelter expands and the occupational therapy department comes together, he plans to focus on trauma. The showers in the shelter are public, and he's trying to figure out how to make that experience more trauma-informed. Shelters are built to be temporary arrangements, but many people have been staying there for a long time. The lack of access to housing is a political problem.

Social aspects like access to safe and stable housing and com-munity spaces, nutritious food, quality education, and equitable healthcare account for 80 percent of a person's health outcomes. Occupational therapy is not covering these areas and is certainly unprepared to address climate change, housing shortages, inflation, homelessness, drug use, and abortion. All real-life shit. As healthcare in the US is based on billing and reimbursements for services, equity work does not fit into the for-profit healthcare infrastructure. The system has to be re-imagined and rebuilt.

Healthcare is inaccessible and unaffordable, and so is higher education, including occupational therapy programs. It's more likely for people who can afford programs to access them. Many graduate occupational therapy programs cost over $60,000 per year, leaving students hundreds of thousands of dollars in debt, with interest constantly accruing, raising that figure each payment period.

The American occupational therapy system can help people reach functional goals but is ineffective in addressing social, cultural, and economic realities. There is much for us to learn from global occupational therapy regarding what the profession can and should address. Adam wants the international occupational therapy community to demand more from the US, hoping to model the successes of global occupational therapy networks. Wherever there are people, there is a need for occupational therapy. Global expansion of the profession with support from rich nations could help with funding and additional resources.

Adam's advice for readers is to shut up and listen to the people we work with. Cultural humility is recognizing that we don't know everything about a culture, even our own. Adam has been Black for 36 years, yet he admits he is not an expert because there are countless Black cultures. We must respect and appreciate all of the diversity in the world and take time to learn about each individual we work with.

There's a barely visible head on the screen as Phin shifts to get comfortable on his dad's lap. I can hear him snoring, quietly. Adam has worked through our talk, caring for his son. It's easy to see that he prioritizes family, even with a heavy workload.

SUGGESTED NEXT STEPS

Reflection: How are you addressing social determinants of health in practice?

Action: Look up histories of segregation in your region. How were people segregated (e.g. based on race, ethnicity, income)? Does that segregation still exist?

Note: As of this publication, Adam is now Director of the Department of Human Services for St. Louis City, where he gets to do similar work at a citywide level.

References

Nardone, A., Casey, J.A., Morello-Frosch, R., Mujahid, M., Balmes, J.R., & Thakur, N. (2020). "Associations between historical residential redlining and current age-adjusted rates of emergency department visits due to asthma across eight cities in California: An ecological study." *The Lancet Planetary Health*, 4(1), doi:10.1016/s2542-5196(19)30241-4.

Steed, R. (2014). "The effects of an instructional intervention on racial attitude formation in occupational therapy students." *Journal of Transcultural Nursing*, 25(4): 403–409, doi:10.1177/1043659614523471.

CHAPTER 9

BRAZIL: Milena Franciely Rodrigues dos Santos

Milena's path to occupational therapy is long and interesting. Born in the countryside of São Paulo in São Carlos, Brazil, Milena Franciely Rodrigues dos Santos is a 22-year-old Brazilian woman studying occupational therapy and working with METUIA, a social occupational therapy program in Brazil, with the core at Universidade Federal de São Carlos (UFSCar). With help from Victor Lemes, an English language teacher who interpreted a previous DisruptOT event, and Felipe Menezes, we arranged a virtual interview with consecutive interpretation. Both Victor and

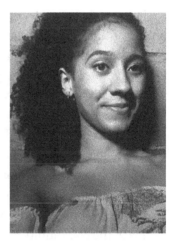

Figure 9.1: Close-up selfie of Milena

Felipe are new to occupational therapy and prepared in advance to learn more and familiarize themselves with the terminology. Before beginning the interview, we take some time to work out the logistics because this is a first for all of us.

We begin the interview with four vignettes sharing one screen. Victor and Felipe are both young Brazilian men with dark hair, mustaches, and goatees, dressed in casual t-shirts, each in well-lit modern-appearing homes in the city of São Carlos. I am a Bengali woman with wavy black and white hair, dressed in a tie-dye blue sweatshirt in my home office in San Francisco, California. Milena, a young Black Brazilian woman, shows up vertically on the screen as she calls in on her phone from her home outside São Carlos. A couple of months ago, her computer stopped working, and she hasn't been able to replace it—a major inconvenience for a student. She's sitting in her blue-walled kitchen with white cabinets and dim lighting, wearing a pink short-sleeved peasant blouse. Her hair is long and black, with coiled curls covering her shoulders.

Victor asks Milena to share her journey to occupational therapy after I ask in English. Excited, she shares in great detail, catching herself to pause and allow Victor to interpret her words back to me. We are all adjusting to this new experience.

In 2015, she was a teenager when her sister invited her to attend programs that METUIA facilitated at her school. She didn't know what occupational therapy was at the time but found the activities interesting and wanted to continue participating. The core of METUIA Network at UFSCar ran these programs. At the time, she didn't consider herself very social, and was mostly shy. She was attending a different school from her sister, and the social occupational therapy project was not offered at her school. These after-school workshops were hands-on and discussion based. Hands-on activities often involved crafts. Discussions covered many topics and some were exclusively for girls. Another program was held in a large youth center open to young people in the community, not just students at the school. She attended all of these and began learning more about occupational therapy.

The girls tended to be more active in discussions, which often centered on their daily routines. Social topics included feminism, sexism, and challenging the idea of women staying at home for domestic responsibilities rather than socializing and being out in the community like men. This was her introduction to these critical topics and occupational therapy.

We pause to ensure everyone's understanding. Victor checks with Felipe to make sure he interpreted Milena's responses accurately. Everything is on track, and we continue with the flow. I ask a question in English, then either Victor or Felipe interprets for Milena. Milena

responds in Portuguese and pauses for translation. Then she continues with her response, which is interpreted for me to understand.
Milena and I are cued by the interpreter gently saying our names so
we know when to continue and recognize the transition in speakers.
Though I cannot interject or stop and ask questions as in a typical
conversation, this is working better than expected. I hardly notice the
pauses as I catch a few words Milena says with my understanding of
Spanish. Her facial expressions say a lot, from comfort, challenges,
relief, and nervousness to nodding in agreement—a universal tell.

The workshops and activities challenged the way of life she was
used to, and the new knowledge gave her a chance to break away
from prior expectations of herself. Now, she could do something and
be someone different. This was an opportunity for herself and other
girls in her community. Captivated by new ways of being, she asked
questions to the faculty involved in these programs. She wanted to
understand why they worked in her community and what they hoped
to do. Her understanding was abstract initially, but as she inquired
more and continued to participate and learn, she understood more
and wanted to be a part of the work.

In 2017, she was ready to study at university and chose occupational
therapy. It was a natural choice after her meaningful experiences
participating in occupational therapy with her community. Entering
the program, she had an idea of what the profession was, but once
she started courses, she realized that it was much broader with many
more areas of focus. Her previous experience with social occupational
therapy, being a local youth, and attending public school gave her the
opportunity to add value as a student occupational therapist.

Milena pauses to think, a little uncertain. With reassurance that
her responses are helpful and well detailed, she continues answering
my question about her current work. This is a new experience for her,
and she is slowly getting comfortable.

METUIA at UFSCar has been offering these services since 2004
in public schools and the community, targeting youth, their families,
schools, and surrounding communities. They aim to improve school
experiences and learning conditions, promote social participation,
and make schools radically inclusive.

Working with METUIA in the neighborhood they grew up in, youth learn about their rights and the inequities they face. The programs run in state public schools in São Carlos in the neighborhoods of Monte Carlo and Jardim Gonzaga. Programs occur during class breaks, in student groups, with teachers, and in school-based clubs. There is a fragile relationship between students and public schools. Students often drop out of school. METUIA's work aims to create new meaning for the students' experiences in school, enabling them to form relationships with and within their schools in a more democratic way, with spaces that allow for valuable discussions, socialization, strategies to promote dynamic learning, and connection with areas of life that are important to them.

Since the start of the COVID-19 pandemic, more students have stopped going to school. Milena's program has been working to search for these students, understand why they stopped going, and find ways to bring them back.

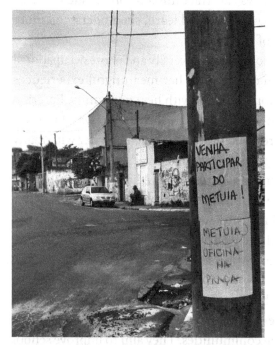

Figure 9.2: METUIA workshop signs on the street to encourage youth to attend. The signs say "Come to METUIA" and "METUIA workshop on the square." (Image from METUIA-UFSCar archive.)

School in Brazil is free and supposed to be mandatory, yet almost three-fifths of the country have fewer than four years of schooling (Encyclopaedia Britannica, n.d.). Poor people are less likely to have access to education. Many students who have dropped out have to work to support their families, with economic conditions worsening since the pandemic. Some are caregivers, while the biggest reason girls stop going to school is because they get pregnant and don't see the point in continuing. High levels of vulnerability in this population make it difficult to succeed and stay in school. METUIA works on addressing the social and cultural barriers that result in them leaving school and keep them from returning.

The social occupational therapy program focuses on individual and collective work to create spaces for open exchange, doing things together, and creating bonds with students. They do this together while paying attention to individual needs, teaching youth to focus on themselves while also creating a community they can depend on. These are democratic spaces for exchange, collaboration, building critical thinking skills, development of autonomy, and self-expression. In addition, they help connect school with the students' realities. The harsh realities of poverty, violence, and trying to survive leave little room to imagine a better or different life. There is an absence of dreams, and part of Milena's role is to help students in the school build plans, to dream again, and find new possibilities.

Prejudice and stigma negatively impact the youths' ability to access social spaces in communities, schools, and outside these places. They also affect participation and keep them from accessing public services, especially poor young people. The program tries to incentivize social participation and convince young people that they have the right to be there as much as anyone else.

The purpose is to widen perspectives and focus on building together while doing interesting and relevant things with them. The program also works with student councils and youth clubs to develop new possibilities for students to be involved in school and their communities, to show them they can do more and be more than the realities they know and are forced into.

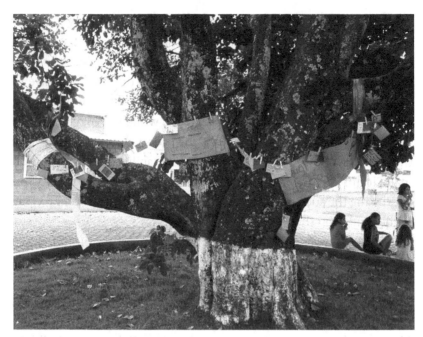

Figure 9.3: Artistic display created from a workshop in the Youth Center on the topic of wishes for the new year. (Image from METUIA-UFSCar archive.)

Milena was born and raised in the neighborhoods she works in. Now, she lives in the adjacent Cidade Aracy. Being a young Black woman from the community and working for the university in her own neighborhood significantly impacts her work and the people she works with. The occupational therapy program has regular internships in these community schools, but being from the community gives her a deeper connection with the people. Her family is still in the neighborhood, so she spends time in the community over the weekends when her presence there goes beyond work. Here, bonds are necessary to build trust with the youth, who don't readily trust people from the outside. She notices this most with the boys, where it is a more prominent barrier to developing bonds and trust. The youth say it's challenging to converse with people from the outside. They "weird them out"—a common sentiment among young people everywhere. It's not necessarily easy for Milena, but their ability to relate to her helps facilitate connection and gain trust so that she can work with them and ease them into opening up.

The neighborhoods she works and lives in are on the city's out-skirts in a very poor region with a lack of infrastructure and resources. It's difficult to access necessary services because of the distance from commercial centers. Jardim Gonzaga is very stigmatized because it's a known place for drug dealing—a daily reality in Brazil and young people's lives. Despite these obstacles, there is a lot of *potência* (power and potential) in the people. Some words don't translate neatly into English; *potência* is one we spend time going back and forth on to ensure that I understand. With the need for this interpretation, it's a lengthy but crucial step. Ultimately, I understand that these youth are resourceful and constantly reinvent themselves and their realities in order to survive.

Victor checks with Felipe to ensure he hasn't missed anything. It's been over an hour, with Victor and Felipe switching interpreter roles every 15 minutes or so. Interpreting requires a significant cognitive load to hear a response in one language and then repeat the words back in another without help from dictionaries or technology. They have to preserve the context and meaning of the original content while adapting culturally specific references for the other person to understand. Multiple layered demands are placed on the interpreter. For a conversation of two and a half hours or more, at least two interpreters are needed to allow for sufficient breaks. However, Victor and Felipe are so interested in learning about social occupational therapy, they each continue listening for their own learning during their minutes off. Milena's phone battery is low. We all take a short break, so she can plug her phone in to complete the interview.

Portuguese is spoken throughout Brazil, though young people commonly use slang. The most common word for occupation is *atividade*, activity, rather than *ocupação*, though she uses different words based on context, area, and approach. Occupation doesn't translate well in Portuguese and can have a negative connotation, as in occupying a person or filling a person with something. Using the word occupation makes it more difficult to explain, while activity is easier and makes more sense. Even in English, occupation can be confusing, commonly mistaken for work or job.

Milena is currently exploring her professional options and enjoys health, education, and the social field. The work she does is individual and collective, aimed at promoting the autonomy of people who cannot fully participate in their daily tasks because of social, physical, or emotional deterrents. Occupational therapists promote engagement, social participation, and access to rights for people and groups, using activities as their tool.

Felipe's connection is bad, and he drops off to reconnect with his phone. Victor resumes interpretation in his place and refers to Milena as Mi to continue. It's sweet to hear him call her by a diminutive, though this is their first meeting.

Despite the challenges in the communities, she enjoys showing the young people the possibilities they could have for their lives. They have dreams and goals but don't know how to achieve them. The most rewarding part of her work is building things collaboratively, watching them create plans, and then reach goals on their own.

I ask if she feels as if she belongs and if occupational therapy is representative of her culture. As this is a complicated and abstract question, I give Victor more details so he can elaborate and explain to Milena. Victor and Milena go back and forth to ensure he understands and can interpret correctly, considering the complexity of her response. Milena responds that she needs to adjust what she has learned in school to fit the community. The theory doesn't always match practice. METUIA goes further by producing its own theories to fit different contexts and communities.

Bringing her perspective and personal experiences is important because she is part of the community and was in the same position as the youth she works with. She has learned from the occupational therapists she worked with in the after-school program that her role is political, ethical, and critical.

Her hopes for occupational therapy in Brazil involve more recognition of the roles of the profession because most people associate occupational therapy with the health sector, and she would like them to understand valuable social aspects. People often mistake the role of social occupational therapists for social workers and psychologists. A recent study she completed with teachers and school administration also reinforced the belief that her work in the schools is associated with social work. Social occupational therapy is misunderstood in Brazil because interventions adapt to the social context and don't neatly fit into a narrow scope or definition. There is even more of a lack of understanding globally despite social occupational therapy's five-decade existence. She wants global occupational therapy to include growth in social and educational fields, as do I.

I ask if she has any advice for readers, and again, she pauses to think through her response, adjusting her hair and looking up to ponder further. She wants readers to recognize that they are working with people from different communities with different experiences and processes. They should welcome and treat people from all communities and focus on guaranteeing their rights and access. How many of us are doing this? The power and actions of the people we work with contribute to a more democratic and political view of healthcare and occupational therapies—described as *potência* (noun) and *potencializar* (verb), to give power, potential, and enhance. She also recommends reading the book *Terapia Ocupacional, Educação e Juventudes* [*Occupational Therapy, Education and Youth*] by Roseli Lopes and Patricia Leme de Oliveira Borba (2022) to help us better understand social occupational therapy.

No more questions remain and I offer her an opportunity to ask me questions. She is curious about my work and who I work with, specifically the demographics. I share that I work in mental health. Less than 3 percent of occupational therapists in the US work in this area (American Occupational Therapy Association, 2015). Because of where I live and the type of services I offer, I only work with adults in my state, and they have diverse identities. I've been an occupational therapist for over ten years, with experience of working in hospitals primarily. I now work for myself and have been using telehealth since the pandemic began.

Milena asks if I have any advice for her career. I tell her she is wise for her age and limited work experience. She understands more about the potential for occupational therapy and connecting with people than many experienced therapists. I encourage her to work with Ana Malfinato, her professor who connected us, to share her work outside Brazil and inspire similar programs in other countries in whichever format she is most comfortable with, publishing or presenting. Smiling wide, showing off her braces, she says she will consider it.

We are over the scheduled time, but everyone is exchanging their appreciation, which takes longer with the need for interpretation. I thank Victor and Felipe for their dedication to this project. We met twice before this interview and exchanged many emails and messages. They both watched videos and read up to understand occupational therapy. Victor started months earlier as he interpreted the April DisruptOT social occupational therapy event. I thank Milena for being open to participating as a student and assure her that her experiences are significant and her words are valuable. She appreciates the opportunity for her work to be visible, though nervous and worried she might not contribute what I expected. We are breaking barriers and doing a first again together—initially, with the presentation from METUIA in Portuguese with simultaneous live English translation, and now with the book and this chapter completed with their help to capture a perspective that would have been overlooked because it did not originate in English.

Now that you have read Milena's story, please take some time to think about occupational therapy in your context. You are invited to engage with DisruptOT on Twitter or at an upcoming free event.

SUGGESTED NEXT STEPS

Reflection: How can/does social occupational therapy fit into your context? How can you incorporate more social aspects into your practice?

Action: Read an article written about social issues or practice in a language that is not your primary language and discuss it with peers.

References

American Occupational Therapy Association (2015). *2015 AOTA salary and workforce survey*. www.aota.org/Education-Careers/Advance-Career/Salary-Workforce-Survey/work-setting-trends-how-to-pick-choose.aspx.

Encyclopaedia Britannica, inc. (n.d.). *Primary and secondary school.* Encyclopaedia Britannica. www.britannica.com/place/Brazil/Primary-and-secondary-school.

Lopes, R. & Leme de Oliveira Borba, P. (2022). *Terapia Ocupacional, Educação e Juventudes [Occupational Therapy, Education and Youth].* São Carlos: EdUFSCar.

CHAPTER 10

THAILAND: Tunchanok Chunvirut

With a delayed internet connection, Tunchanok Chunvirut, a Thai woman with long, straight, black hair, turns her camera off while speaking with me from her home in Bangkok, Thailand. Originally from Kamphaeng Phet, a town between two major cities, Tunchanok moved to Chiang Mai to study and later to the capital city of Bangkok to work. An occupational therapist for ten years with experience in mental health settings, she works at the Somdet Chaopraya Institute of Psychiatry, where occupational therapy started in Thailand.

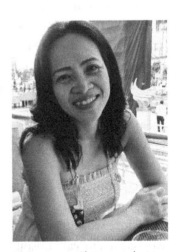

Figure 10.1: Close-up photo of Tunchanok sitting outside

In college, she had to select a course, and without knowing what occupational therapy was, she chose it because the course description interested her. In Thailand, you can change your course of studies after one year in university. If it's not a good fit, switching to another program is possible. Though she still didn't understand what occupational therapy was through the first year, she was happy with the faculty and decided to stay. At the time of her studies, there was only one occupational therapy program at Chiang Mai University.

Currently, three programs are available, with options to enter the profession with a bachelor's or master's degree. In addition, there will soon be a PhD option.

When Tunchanok was a student, all of her classes were offered in Thai. The English language was not as popular as it is now, and there was not as much Western influence in the country. Thailand is one of the few countries in Asia that was not a European colony, and this preserved its local culture and language. Occupational therapy textbooks were in English, so her professors translated them into Thai to teach students. Adaptation was also required for culture and context, as they were written for Western readers and did not match Thai occupations and lifestyles.

Many recommendations were too costly for the average household or facility. For instance, sensory integration was taught to be incorporated through the use of sensory rooms with expensive equipment. This was, and still is, not affordable for hospitals and other facilities. Instead, they adapted what they learned about sensory equipment to include outdoor environments like gardens with water features and the use of rocks, soil, grass, and plants, with various textures, smells, and sensory components. In place of a sensory swing, they placed old tires on trees to make swings. These are sensible adaptations, given that equipment in hospitals isn't available in homes. These options are far more available to the average household.

Before working at the government-funded Institute, Tunchanok worked at a private hospital. Private hospitals in Thailand are funded by self-payment or private insurance, whereas government-funded hospitals are free for locals to access. In the free hospitals, people who are not Thai citizens have to pay for services.

Somdet Chaopraya Institute of Psychiatry offers both inpatient and outpatient services. The majority of patients, almost 80 percent, are residents of Bangkok. Other patients are likely to have been in the city for work when they needed psychiatric care.

Inpatient stays at the Institute are usually one month long, with occupational therapy services beginning a week or two before discharge. After discharge, most patients will return home to their families. Part of the occupational therapist's role is to prepare the patient and their family for returning home and prevent relapse through education on signs and symptoms, when to seek early help, and how to provide support at home.

About a month after discharge, a nurse visits patients' homes to assess how they are doing. If recommended, an occupational therapist will do a home visit and provide additional support. Follow-up phone calls are more common for occupational therapists on Tunchanok's team, with a limited number of staff for visiting every home.

For outpatient care, much of her focus is on vocational training. Patients are taught various handicrafts that the Institute purchases and sells in the hospital gift shop. Various job opportunities are available at the hospital gift shop, an on-site and local coffee shop chain, and other businesses that partner with the Institute.

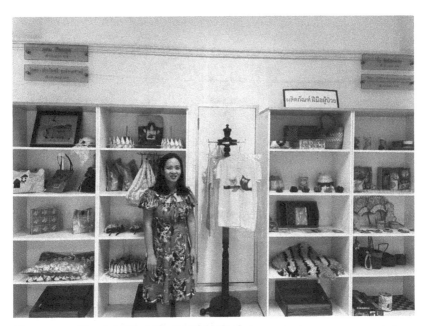

Figure 10.2: Tunchanok at the facility gift shop, featuring handicrafts made by patients

The coffee shop in the facility doubles as a site for training. Several locations throughout Bangkok employ patients. The coffee shop business is a social enterprise committed to supporting patients to succeed with employment and has been working with the hospital for almost eight years, one of its longest partnerships. The company built a fully functional location on-site to train new staff who happen to be hospital patients. They send supervising staff in to prepare to support workers with mental health conditions. This training includes supporting these workers in maintaining their work roles and looking for signs and symptoms that warrant professional support or medical care. Occupational therapists train and support all staff and managers, including workers with mental illness.

Other companies work with the Institute, though none are as involved as the coffee shop business. Additional business relationships are difficult to maintain. When training and placements are unsuccessful, some opt to discontinue the partnership rather than receive additional support and training to make it work.

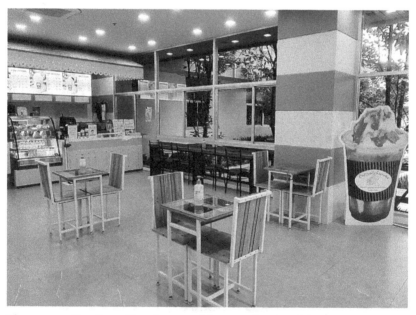

Figure 10.3: On-site coffee shop used for vocational training

The facility director is very supportive of the occupational therapy team and is responsible for establishing these partnerships. The hospital is invested in reducing stigma in the community and helping patients be active and accepted members of the local community and wider society. Work is a meaningful way to ensure they can thrive, live independently, and demonstrate potential for inclusion. In the country, there is a belief that people with mental illness are burdens and with a lot of poverty in the city, earning a steady income is essential to surviving.

Education plays a significant role in occupational therapy and mental health facilities like the Institute. Tunchanok and her colleagues also train staff at smaller hospitals that do not have occupational therapy, and offer education to family members.

Five occupational therapists work at the Institute, and there is a need for more. With over 1300 therapists in the country, there aren't enough to cover all 77 provinces and almost 70 million people in Thailand. With help from the Thai Occupational Therapy Association, it has been easier to have occupational therapy recognized throughout the country. The profession is well established with three educational programs. There is a strong presence of occupational therapists in mental health settings, with the profession beginning in this area of care. Physical rehabilitation is another common practice setting.

Like many regions, occupational therapy is often confused with physical therapy. Most hospitals have physical therapy, but only hospitals in major cities have occupational therapy. Most Thai occupational therapists stay in the country because family is an integral part of their culture, and they don't want to be far from them despite being able to make more money abroad. Their family bonds are more important than money.

Family is important in Thailand. Several generations often live in the same household, making it common for young adults to remain at home through college and professional life. Family members help take care of the elderly, young children, ill, and disabled members.

Reintegrating patients returning home and into the community after discharge can be a major challenge. Families are sometimes afraid they may be unable to manage symptoms, and members of average families have to work, so no one is at home to support the patient. Some families will return patients to the hospital even when they are stable and don't have significant enough symptoms to require hospitalization because they are worried about the reoccurrence of a mental health crisis. Part of their education is teaching the family to recognize early signs before a full relapse.

Some families are unwilling to accept the person back home after discharge from the hospital. While some are worried they might not be able to offer proper support, many are simply too poor. They have to work and cannot take time off to care for or stay with the patient, so they are left at home alone. Poor families are less likely to accept patients back home. Tunchanok finds it painfully sad when patients want to return home but cannot. Some don't understand why and she has to console them and explain the situation. Families are offered the choice of returning home or help with a placement in supportive housing.

Supportive group homes are an alternative to returning home. However, there is rarely space available. These homes are connected to the hospital; staff help administer medication and transition patients back to the hospital if needed. They are housed, fed, cared for, and can access treatment. While waiting for a placement, patients are stuck in the hospital.

Homelessness is not common in Thailand because of family structures, and the government provides housing for people, so it is rare to see anyone living on the street. Furthermore, the government pays for these housing alternatives.

There is a lot of stigma and shame around mental illness and seeking help. People are worried about admitting they have a mental illness and others finding out. There is a perception that someone experiencing mental illness is weak and unable to get over their symptoms. The stigma is improving with investments and public campaigns. Recently, a Thai superstar promoted the psychiatric hospital to normalize seeking support. Campaigns like this are becoming more popular in Thailand. Younger generations are more open to talking about mental health. However, sensationalized news reports of mentally ill people being aggressive don't help.

Despite the challenges, Tunchanok loves what she does and has a lot of fun in her daily interactions with patients. Cooking is one of the most popular activities because they all get to eat afterwards. Bua Loy is a typical Thai dessert they make together with flour, coconut milk, and sugar. Rolling the dough in the palm of your hands is one of the steps and incorporates soothing sensory input that many patients enjoy. Tunchanok's work is rewarding, and she feels valued. There are occasions when patients can become aggressive, and she has been hit before, but the positive moments are more impressive. Patients typically enjoy occupational therapy the most. The activities bring them joy and entertain them while in the hospital. They get to be themselves and not worry about anything else during those moments.

Thai is spoken with patients unless they are foreign, which is rare. The Thai term for occupational therapy, นักกิจกรรมบำบัด (*nuk-kij-ja-kam-bumbud*), translates to activity therapy.

She describes Bangkok as sunny and feeling like summer all year round. Even in the winter, it's not cold. People are polite, respectful, and humble. Unfortunately, this also means that they hide their feelings and are more worried about making other people happy, keeping their problems to themselves. They only want the good to be seen and hide the other parts of themselves, which can be problematic in getting support they could benefit from. Tunchanok's job is to teach people about their emotions and how to express them, how to voice their needs, and set boundaries. The social aspect of culture and pleasing people is strong. She shares a familiar example of people having difficulty saying no to friends regarding drug use, which complicates addressing and supporting substance misuse.

She has seen mental health occupational therapy in Hong Kong and Malaysia and recognizes many similarities in the field, although policies and government support differ. For example, in Hong Kong, there is much more support and more opportunities for patients because the government gives monetary help while they are in the hospital. Not only is the hospitalization paid for, but in some cases, patients receive money to offset their salary while they are there. In Thailand, many people can't return to the hospital after they relapse or when they need care because they can't afford it. Although locals don't have to pay for medical care, they have to pay to travel to the hospital, and this expense can be a barrier.

There aren't any occupational therapy textbooks specific to the Asian context yet, so everything she learned had to be adapted to the local context and culture. Especially in mental health, we must understand a person's culture and perspectives, otherwise we won't understand them or their needs. With steps taken to understand a person, it is easier to build trust, which is essential to receiving the best care. Taking time to understand people results in the patient's greater willingness to work together and accept care, and makes interventions more applicable for better outcomes. The context and environment are equally crucial to understanding a person's needs.

Tunchanok hopes that Thailand will have enough occupational therapists to work in every hospital one day. Some occupational therapists work in schools, though most are in urban health centers, which the rural areas don't have access to. She also wants more global connections for the profession so we can learn from each other, share ideas, and better adapt to various cultures and contexts. These types of exchanges will not only offer a sharing of best practices but an opportunity to learn about each other's cultures. This is even easier now with virtual connections.

The mission of DisruptOT is to connect people worldwide and offer them free education about global occupational therapies, healthcare, and critical concerns. Free opportunities make access possible for anyone, especially those in low-income countries who might not be able to attend expensive international conferences.

Tunchanok's advice for readers is to understand people and their cultures before considering treatment options. This will help interventions be more relevant and make it more likely that they will want to work with us. She believes this book will give people some insight into the diversity of occupational therapies from several world perspectives, including introductions to their cultures and contexts. It is hoped that this will promote interest and understanding of people from different countries, cultures, and environments.

SUGGESTED NEXT STEPS

Reflection: What is the state of mental healthcare in your region? How can occupational therapy include mental health interventions in settings that are not considered psychosocial?

Action: Look up mental healthcare in three countries you have never visited and don't know much about. What do they have in common? What are some differences?

CHAPTER 11

ICELAND: Ósk Sigurdardottir

Ósk Sigurdardottir is a 47-year-old Icelandic woman with dark hair and blue eyes. She lives with her partner, four children, and dog Simba just outside Reykjavik, the capital of Iceland. An occupational therapist with formal education and experience in various roles, she studied in Denmark just before Iceland started its first occupational therapy program the same year.

When she graduated high school in 1996, there were no occupational therapy programs in the country. She took a career test to decide on her future studies, which recommended three pro-

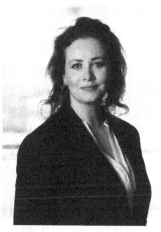

Figure 11.1: Close-up photo of Ósk standing in front of a window

fessions. One was occupational therapy. Not having a clue what it was, she looked into it and found a job as an occupational therapy assistant at a local rehabilitation center. At the time, it wasn't common for recent graduates to take a year off, but Ósk didn't want to rush into the big decision. Working in the rehabilitation center for a year, she fell in love with occupational therapy. A self-described doer who likes to find solutions, she readily made connections with patients and helped them find solutions to everyday problems. The hands-on nature of the role locked it in for her, and she moved to Denmark to get her bachelor's degree in occupational therapy, where it was well established.

Soon after she started, a program opened in Akureyri, Iceland. There were only a few occupational therapists in Iceland at the time, even fewer with master's or PhD degrees, so it took some time to come together. Before the local program opened, most occupational therapists studied in nearby Nordic countries, some going as far as the UK, Australia, and the US.

It is more common nowadays for newly graduated students to take a year off before starting university. Upper secondary school, also known as high school, used to be four years and is now three. Students graduate a year earlier at 19 years old and take advantage of the extra year to explore work and the world. In Ósk's experience, this was more common for her classmates in Denmark.

There is less pressure in Nordic countries to go straight into university or find a career. Time spent with family and friends and experiencing other areas in life is highly valued. The social system allows for this possibility, with the government offering free funds that do not require repayment in many Nordic countries, while repayment is required in Iceland. Student loans are an option, with delayed payments and low interest rates, and childcare is subsidized. This makes higher education more accessible and affordable, even allowing for a career change later in life. Compare this to the US, with expensive childcare and private universities charging $50,000 or more per year for occupational therapy programs, and high interest rates on student loans that far exceed local salaries. There is no room to switch careers, as loans can take 20 years or more to pay off.

When Ósk graduated, there were around 200 occupational therapists in the Denmark, and now there are nearly 500. The profession is growing, though not everyone knows what occupational therapy is yet.

She studied and completed her internships in Denmark. It was a three-year program with 24 weeks of clinical practice, and she did one clinical placement in Iceland. Fundamental courses were similar, but the emphasis on clinical practice was greater in Denmark than in Iceland, which helped her connect theory to practice.

With similar cultures in both countries, Denmark is more advanced in rehabilitation and psychiatry in first-line services in the community, schools, and hospitals. Before someone goes to hospital for admission, they meet with someone from their municipality. When they are ready to be discharged, there is another meeting with someone from the community who can connect them to local services. There is always a link to ongoing support, with consistent communication between services. She hopes this will be replicated in Iceland.

With fewer occupational therapists in Iceland, she had more autonomy in developing programs. Denmark offers more comprehensive training with more therapists and a long-established profession. As a result, she was better prepared for practice with Danish training. The Icelandic programs are newer, and, based on her experience of taking student interns, they are less well prepared.

In her first year, she studied adult psychiatry in Denmark in the middle of the woods. Patients were permitted to go outside and forage for berries, mushrooms, and other foods to prepare inside. She enjoyed the program so much that it became her first workplace after graduation.

When she returned home to Iceland, she took her first job in child and adolescent psychiatry in the only hospital where children could access this type of care. There were only two occupational therapists there at the time, so she played a significant part in shaping the department and proving that her function was essential. She remained there for ten years, with five as the head of the department.

After this, Ósk worked in various leadership roles in settings where occupational therapists aren't typically found. Using her professional skills and additional education, she improved processes in the Chief Executive Officer's (CEO) office at the National Hospital and helped develop large-scale housing projects, designing the environment to promote health, for example by adding gardens. She was also President of the Iceland Occupational Therapy Association for six years.

In a culmination of her leadership and clinical journey, she now uses all of the skills she's built as the CEO of Sjálfsbjörg lsh (National Federation of Physically Disabled People in Iceland), and the Vice President of Römpum upp Ísland (Ramp up Iceland). The National Federation advocates for the rights of disabled people. They build accessible apartments, ensure that young people can study and access universities, help disabled people find work and participate in daily life, and work on various projects to make Iceland more accessible. She also teaches innovation to occupational therapy and master's students in health sciences at the University of Akureyri.

I was curious about her myriad leadership roles that stray from the typical occupational therapy professional path. She laughs as she shares her rich educational background, going through a long list of degrees and her inspiration to pursue them. Her account is consistently structured and well prepared, as she runs through her educational background, checking her notes occasionally to ensure nothing is missed.

The therapeutic communication skills she learned at university and in practice weren't cutting it for the children she worked with. With a deep love for art, she moved to Barcelona to get a master's in art therapy to bridge this gap and add to what she could offer at the hospital. Then, feeling that her leadership skills could use improvement, she got a master's in project management. Taking a Scrum course in this program, she used her occupational therapy knowledge to build the TravAble mobile application, helping travelers find accessible services and places to visit in 34 countries.

After this degree, she went to work in the hospital CEO's office, helping people and departments, and solving different problems and improving processes. Finding an exciting innovation program and constantly pushing herself to learn, do, and be more, she studied at Oxford University and rounded out her education with a master's in business administration, becoming the CEO of the National Federation of Physically Disabled People in Iceland. She was fortunate to have access to this education, some support from the country's social systems to pay for school in the region, and help with childcare, and these opportunities propelled her career even further.

She teaches a required entrepreneurship course in the occupational therapy program. Entrepreneurship in occupational therapy is rare in Iceland, a country with socialized medicine. There is typically more incentive to be an entrepreneur in privately funded healthcare. This course focuses on service and product offerings, marketing, hiring, and funding. Ultimately, students have to present their new company. Aside from creating a business, the entrepreneurial mindset is about seeing a gap, finding a way to address it, and fostering a problem-solving philosophy. We ask patients to adapt; we should be able to as well.

Instead of explaining, she plays a video of Halli, Haraldur Ingi Þorleifsson (Haraldur Thorleifsson), founder of Römpum upp Reykjavík (Ramp up Reykjavik) and Römpum upp Ísland (Ramp up Iceland), sharing the progress of their project. He tells his personal story as a wheelchair user for 20 years. When his family went for a walk in downtown Reykjavik, steps separated him from his family when going into shops and restaurants. With the organization, he set a goal for 100 ramps in one year in downtown Reykjavik. Their model includes ramps being free of charge to store owners, handling permits for them, building permanent structures, and making ramps beautiful by fitting them into existing environments. At the time of the video, they had built 101 ramps in eight months, surpassing the goal and leaving funds available to build more. Because Ramp up Reykjavik went so well, they started a bigger project. Ramp up Iceland started in March 2022 with the goal of building 1500 ramps all over Iceland. By December 2022, 350 ramps had been built.

Before and after images of storefronts show almost invisible new ramps, matching pavers, making entrances flush with the sidewalk. They used simple messaging to get everyone involved, from politicians, businesses, and building owners to the press and the local public. They did such a great job that people contacted them to participate. They brought to life the idea of community, with everyone working together to overcome barriers. The plans are all open source for anyone in the world to access.

Occupation in Icelandic is *iðjuþjálfun*, meaning practice work. Ósk explains the occupational therapist's role as enabling people to participate in the activities of daily life—things they want, need, or expect to do. It's about finding solutions to have a meaningful everyday life, enhance ability, or modify the environment. When working, she mainly speaks Icelandic and occasionally Danish. With more immigrants moving to the country, recently she has been using more

English. All Icelandic children learn Icelandic, English, and Danish in school. There is also an option to learn Spanish, French, or German as an additional language. With popular culture, television, and film, English is spoken throughout the country now.

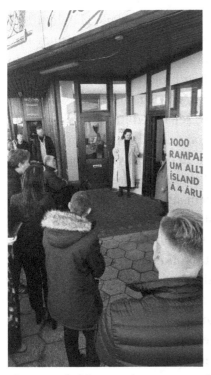

Figure 11.2: Ribbon cutting ceremony for Römpum upp Ísland

Serving the entire country in her roles, Ósk sees the whole country as her community. Her work ensures that everyone, regardless of where they live, can participate in whatever they want to do. The biggest challenges she faces are funding, older inaccessible build- ings, and bureaucracy. The NGOs she works with in the country are collaborating and co-competing. They work together on political advocacy because they are small and do better in numbers to convince politicians to take on issues and put solutions into law. At the same time, they are competing for donations.

The capital city, Reykjavik, has the majority of services, and the smaller municipalities have fewer resources. Getting them to offer the same services and access she is working toward is a more significant challenge. Much of her work is dependent on volunteer support, but it's getting harder to find young volunteers and as older ones age they aren't able to be as involved.

In community building, we can't expect people to trust or accept us, so we show up consistently to prove our intentions. This takes time and effort. In addition to regular phone calls and virtual meetings, Ósk travels around the country to be more visible and available to the people and organizations she works with.

With the National Federation, she works alongside the Icelandic Tourist Board. They look at hotels, restaurants, and tourist destinations around the country from an accessibility standpoint and educate staff and owners on disability inclusion in their spaces.

She loves fostering and being part of the community, never understanding why some people can participate while others can't. The barriers were created, so we can tear them down. It just requires money, time, effort, and people.

There's a common saying in Iceland, *þetta reddast*, which roughly translates to we will find a solution and finish this undertaking. With a rich fishing history, Icelanders are known to be headstrong and work hard, and long hours, to get things done. There is not a lot of hierarchy in Iceland. Regular people can speak with national government leaders. For example, the national hospital's CEO sits in the same space as everyone else, without a private office. Humility can help move things forward and get people to work well together because they are valued equally. People are more open to working together without social hierarchy. Although it's not completely idyllic, as Ósk notes that overall income inequality is increasing in the country, despite gender equality improving and the gender wage gap slowly closing.

Ósk wants more occupational therapists to provide preventative care in her home country. Services in schools and more community care options will help people before they are in crisis and at the point of needing to go to the hospital. Preventive care, and families and communities helping each other will save lives and money in the long run. She wants occupational therapists to be unafraid to try different things, and she is mentoring people to do just that.

Through her experience with the World Federation of Occupational Therapists and the Council of Occupational Therapists for the European Countries, Ósk visited different hospitals and met clinicians in other parts of the world. She found that there are a lot of common challenges. We are all working toward the same goals.

Ósk's experiences are in stark contrast to mine. In the US, people in locked psychiatric units require permission to go outside to walled outdoor spaces. They are not healing environments. Often compared to incarceration, these spaces don't always enhance health. The Nordic consideration for outdoor spaces, sun exposure, human interaction, nature, and wildlife contributes to healing. In Iceland, there is support to return to work, while in the US, there is no mandated maternity leave or support and no guaranteed healthcare for parents or babies. Social support, or lack thereof, can dictate what occupational therapy looks like in a country. Health risks increase without a system of support or community involvement, and engaging in occupations becomes more problematic.

Occupational therapy is political. Necessary equipment, regulations, and health insurance are getting written out of insurance policies. For example, there was a local issue with grab bars no longer being covered, so Ósk helped write an article and met with social ministers to explain why this was a bad idea. People were falling and breaking their hips and spending time in hospital. This was costing significantly more than paying for the grab bars which would prevent falls.

Though more common in other Nordic countries, research is increasing in Iceland. Ósk wants more regional textbooks, research, and political involvement. With shared heritage, values, and culture, it makes sense to work with nearby countries and learn from each other—something she is doing in her national roles.

She hopes there will soon be a master's program in Iceland, once several occupational therapists have received a PhD. There are currently six or seven in the process of doing so. This might help with salary increases. It is a predominantly woman-dominated profession, with a lower salary than physical therapy, which consists primarily of men, with many in private practice.

Globally, she wants occupational therapy to be a valued and better-respected profession that shares our work internationally. As a result, we can be everywhere, working with anyone and providing value anywhere.

This book is about how things work in other countries and what we might consider trying. Even though things are done a certain way, we can still try something different and see if we can improve things. This is the entrepreneur's mindset—what Ósk wants all occupational therapists to have.

She comes from a privileged country and has to remind herself that not everyone has access to the same resources. Her advice for readers is to be open and to ask questions, not be judgmental. Diverse groups allow us to learn from each other, so we should be open and honest if we don't know about someone's culture and be curious to learn more.

SUGGESTED NEXT STEPS

Reflection: How accessible is the area you live in? What features can be improved to promote universal access?

Action: For the next three days, track every place you visit or watch on television and note what is not accessible and how it can be made more accessible.

CHAPTER 12

BOTSWANA: Lady Gofaone Modise

Lady Gofaone Modise is a Motswana (native to Botswana) occupational therapist working as a case manager in Gaborone, Botswana. Originally an officer with the Botswana Motor Vehicle Accident Fund, a public organization for people injured in road crashes, she now works there in a management position. Their mission is "to enhance the quality of life by promoting road safety, compensating, rehabilitating and supporting those affected by road crashes."

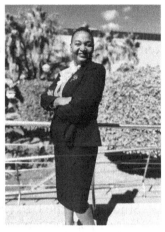

Figure 12.1: Lady standing outside

Her role aligns with her occupational therapy training to get people back to their occupations and everyday lives. Case management begins in the acute care setting in the hospital and continues with any medical care needed, including rehabilitation and return to work programs. She works with healthcare providers to ensure that funds are authorized and accessible when the claimant needs them. This level of coverage is only available to those who have sustained motor vehicle-related injuries. Though she doesn't practice as a traditional therapist anymore, she uses those skills in various ways to help people recovering from injuries throughout their rehabilitation journey.

Growing up, Lady was good at sciences and even won a biology prize in high school. She wanted to study abroad, which back then typically required a pre-bachelor's degree at the University of Botswana before further education abroad. In her first year of university, she continued to enjoy and excel in science courses and knew she wanted to help people, so she thought that health sciences would be a good fit. At a local career fair, a Motswana occupational therapist who trained in Australia and currently works in British Columbia discussed occupational therapy as a career choice. It resonated with what she wanted to do to help people.

Lady shadowed this occupational therapist at her hospital job to understand more about what she did. At the time, there were only about five Batswana (natives of Botswana) occupational therapists, ten across the country though not all from the country. That made her even more interested in what seemed like a rare specialty. In her second year of college, she observed another occupational therapist in a mining town, offering more than the typical hospital-based government services like pediatrics, return to work, and advocacy. Here she realized the breadth of practice options. After her second year at the University of Botswana, she had to choose a profession and decided on occupational therapy.

Studying in the UK, US, or South Africa is most common. She studied at Cardiff University in the UK. The program used problem-based learning, so she was taught to be a critically thinking occupational therapist who looks at problems and solves them for each context. The approach focused on understanding the person and what is important to them. This made it easier for her to take what she learned and apply it in the local context.

At the time, most occupational therapists in the country were from Kenya. Currently, there are about 30 practicing occupational therapists in Botswana, with only 22 being Batswana. Most work in hospital settings, while four, a significant portion of the country's therapists, work for the Fund in distinctive non-clinical capacities, and another four in private practice.

Since 2021, Botswana has been an associate member of the World Federation of Occupational Therapists (WFOT). There are no occupational therapy programs in the country yet, so people must study abroad. A local university is working on starting a program, which the Botswana Occupational Therapy Association and the Health Professions Council are also involved with.

As a case manager, Lady wanted to learn more about healthcare management, not just the clinical side, so she pursued a master's in business administration in the healthcare management stream. However, her heart was still in occupational therapy, and she was passionate about return to work, especially after seeing how road crashes can disrupt people's lives, and how with advocacy and support they can get back to work. So, now she is pursuing a PhD in return to work and developing an operational framework for people receiving loss-of-income benefits with the University of Pretoria in South Africa. This is an income benefit for people who lose employment or the ability to earn an income. This may be the end of the road for many people. She believes that there are many possibilities to return to work in a coordinated way and is using her distinct work experience to help more people.

An occupational therapist for 12 years, with ten in her current position, she is also the Vice President of the Botswana Occupational Therapy Association and the Chairperson of the Botswana Health Professions Council Occupational Therapy Board.

In her association and board roles, she advocates through social media and local media (radio and television) to bring awareness to the profession. Many areas in the country are underserved, and with very few occupational therapists, they can only work in a few hospitals and facilities. She is privileged to work in an organization that allows her to facilitate the occupational therapy role, necessary equipment, and services that aren't always available in these traditional healthcare spaces. As a result, clients receive better care than most people in the country and receive benefits equitably, regardless of their income and instead based on need.

Anyone involved in a vehicle accident in Botswana is eligible for services, and she works with people around the country from the capital city of Gaborone. In a remarkable system, a fuel levy pays for these services, allowing for generous benefits for anyone who qualifies. Services and length of coverage are based on the type of claim. There are limited claims of up to 300,000 pula and unlimited claims of up to 1,000,000 pula, almost ten times the country's average annual salary, to cover all of their medical needs. These are significant amounts, considering what life would be like without these critical services that the average person could not access or afford if they had significant medical needs.

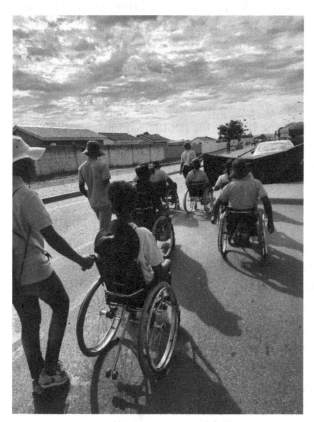

Figure 12.2: A wheelchair walk organized for clients by the Fund

Government-sponsored healthcare might include longer wait times and additional challenges, such as less funding. In contrast, the Fund pays for whatever the clients need. It's comparable to working in private services where there are fewer barriers and superior care, but where only the privileged few can afford it. But, Lady can provide high-quality services to her clients regardless of their income, and get them what they need.

There are many things she loves about her work, and she believes it's one of the best places she can work in Botswana as an occupational therapist. Clients with catastrophic injuries who didn't believe they could return to work have managed to do so. When she sees them successfully using assistive devices and returning to the community, doing what they love and what is purposeful to them, it brings her joy. Some people aren't comfortable returning to work or public spaces after significant injuries. She shares a story of one client who returned to school to study fashion design and has since started working as a fashion designer, designing for the community and herself. One of her biggest wins was advocating for a client to be fitted with a myoelectric prosthesis, an artificial limb controlled by input from electrical signals generated by muscles in the residual limb, when they were still new. Some clients speak at the organization's caregiver training seminars and conferences and other disability arenas and advocate for disability policies. Occasionally, she sees clients in the community returning to their lives, school, and work. The best part of her job is seeing clients flourishing in the community.

Setswana and English are the most commonly spoken languages in Botswana. Depending on the client's language preference, Lady uses either of these languages and interpreters for different tribal languages, or sign language.

Describing occupation or what occupational therapy is, is a common problem. In Setswana, she explains it as *go dira*, to do. Many people think it is only about paid employment, so she explains that she looks at all activities that they do, from waking up to going to bed, and elaborates on different activities they might want or need to do that are meaningful and bring value and purpose to their life. Often, it's easier for her to ask people what they really wish they could do and explain from that perspective. Other terms commonly used in practice are *go itshetsa* (engagement in economic activities) and *ditiro tsa gago tsa tsatsi le letsatsi* (activities of daily living).

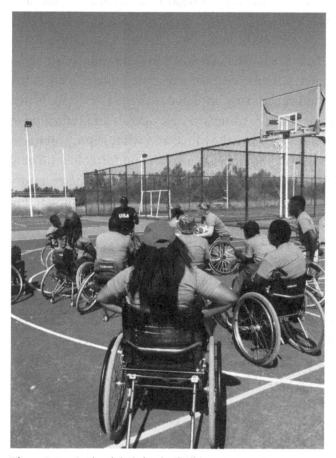

Figure 12.3: A wheelchair basketball event

Botswana is a peaceful country, something Lady no longer takes for granted. In 2016, she was part of the Mandela Washington Fellowship for Young African Leaders, a program initiated by President Obama for academic leadership and training. She was placed at Ohio State University, where she met many young African leaders. Listening to their stories of war and struggles in their home countries, she realized how fortunate she was. She was sponsored by the government to complete undergraduate education, and her country's education and healthcare are subsidized. Hearing stories of the hardships many women faced, she could not help but compare it to the safety and many opportunities afforded to her, especially as a woman. Married with two boys, her husband and those around her support her ambitions.

In 2018, she was in Mozambique as part of a fellowship and witnessed the aftermath of natural disasters and floods while researching inclusive education in schools. Grateful for what is available in Botswana, she also knows there is room for improvement, like most countries.

In her experiences abroad, she noticed that high-income countries have more resources for healthcare and elaborate interventions. The level of funding and research can drive change and policies, allowing for a more competitive and evolving practice. She is working on that now with help from the Elizabeth Casson Trust, which is funding part of her doctoral sponsorship. She could also attend the WFOT congress online because of their award, and learn from African scholars and clinicians.

When she attends international conferences, she looks at how many African people are in the room and how many women are represented. This representation signifies belonging and potential for her and women like her. When she sees accomplished African occupational therapists like Tecla Mlambo and Tongai Chichaya, she wants to know them and sees herself in them. These are people whose articles she wants to read, quote, and cite because their research is relevant to her work. She wants to promote opportunities for improvements, education, and research to other Africans so they can reach the next level, as she did.

As we discuss her experiences and her sense of belonging in her home country, she mentions that she doesn't feel Black in Botswana. She isn't excluded because of her race, unlike in the US, where the Black Lives Matter movement grew out of the need to dismantle systemic racism, injustices, and inequities robbing Black people of their lives at a greater rate. I'm forced to pause. Her casual message has a deeper meaning. She is safe in Botswana and can live her life without worrying about how she will be treated because of her skin color and heritage—a peace that does not apply to all Africans.

There are only a few books with Afrocentric approaches in occupational therapy written by Africans, which means that the majority of texts come from a Western context. A common concern is income and food security, rather than Western priorities like leisure. Though an African contextual occupational therapy book will not solve these problems, it could offer African solutions to African problems.

Lady has big hopes for occupational therapy in Botswana. Once the occupational therapy program in the country is up and running, it will have a significant impact because, currently, the numbers are too low. For there to be a substantial change, there will need to be occupational therapists in every district, city, and town. People are traveling thousands of miles to access services in big cities. She wants occupational therapy services to be affordable and accessible for every Motswana. This is why she is doing her PhD in occupational therapy and returning to her professional roots.

Her advice for readers is to understand the context, culture, beliefs, and what's important to the people we work with. Practice empathy first to find relevant, meaningful, interesting, and encouraging interventions. Respect cultural values and personal beliefs and let those drive interventions and practice.

She encourages readers to put themselves out there and reach for opportunities they are afraid of. We need to read and familiarize ourselves with things that put us out of our comfort zones—challenge ourselves beyond what we think we can do.

Now that the interview has ended, Lady turns her camera on. It was an unexpectedly long work day, and she had worked out just before we met. Someone who takes pride in her presentation, Lady is accustomed to wearing lipstick and dressing up. She doesn't want to be recorded without her usual preparation but agrees to take a selfie screenshot with me. Wearing a casual black t-shirt, she poses with a slight head tilt showing off her natural face, short hair, closed mouth smile, and ring on her finger, in front of a lime green wall in her office.

SUGGESTED NEXT STEPS

Reflection: What are you grateful for in your region? What can be improved in your region?

Action: What does representation mean to you? For the next three days, notice who is in each room you enter or show or film you watch. Do they represent you? What representation is lacking?

Note: As of this publication, Lady now works for the Botswana Medical Aid Society as a Claims Manager.

CHAPTER 13

TRINIDAD AND TOBAGO:
Khamara-Lani Tarradath

A self-described island girl, Khamara-Lani Tarradath is a Trinbagonian woman and occupational therapist in Trinidad and Tobago, the southernmost country in the Caribbean consisting of the two main islands and a chain of 21 additional islands, each with distinct and shared cultures. She is a Caribbean woman with long black locs, effusive expressions, and a prominent smile. Her grandmother was the descendant of one of the wives of an enslaver. Her grandfather, Tarradath Maharajh, is of Nepalese descent. In 1945, he had to change his name around to appear more Christian

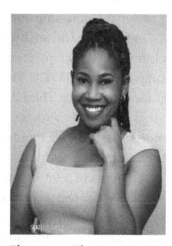

Figure 13.1: Close-up photo of Khamara-Lani

to teach in the country and reassure his dark-skinned wife of African descent, who faced backlash for carrying such a distinctly East Indian name. Raised with Hindu and Christian influences with mixed heritage, she is representative of the country's rich and complex cultures.

As an occupational therapist, she assumes many practical and leadership roles. She has two clinical jobs and holds the position of Chair of the Trinidad and Tobago Occupational Therapy Association (TTOTA) and the Occupational Therapy and Speech Language Pathology Board, the regulatory board for the professions in the country.

Always interested in medicine, she thought she wanted to be a doctor. Then, one day, her mother heard an occupational therapist on the radio, Priya Gomes, describing her fascinating work, which she only vaguely knew about. Her mother shared the details, and she met with Priya and began volunteering, recognizing on the first day that this was the profession for her. Priya is still her mentor.

At the time, there was no local occupational therapy program. People would have to go abroad and find a way to make it work once they returned home. There was no clear path to becoming a working occupational therapist, with limited government positions and support. But, her family was supportive, and she knew that being an occupational therapist would be valuable in caring for her grandmother with Alzheimer's, who has recently passed away. She received a national scholarship and went to North Florida to study.

In 2016, the University of the Southern Caribbean introduced an occupational therapy program, developed by Dr. Lesley Garcia and supported by TTOTA. This program has seen about 21 Caribbean students graduate. This is the first master's level occupational therapy program in the English-speaking Caribbean. With this program being more accessible, the number of practicing occupational therapists in the country is growing.

There were a lot of barriers before the local program opened. Khamara-Lani learned about the profession by chance. Then she had to complete an in-person interview with the program in Florida and was brought in for additional questioning five times when applying for a student visa. Her visa expired the day her program ended, leaving no cushion for delays, which is common with limited fieldwork placements in the US. There were issues with the scholarship paying her tuition, and gaining work experience cost her additional funds, including applying for a work visa. Looking back, she isn't sure how she overcame all the obstacles.

Undergraduate education is subsidized in Trinidad and Tobago. Master's programs are self-funded, with limited scholarships available. The occupational therapy master's program is longer and more expensive that the average local master's programs. Only those who can afford the tuition and additional time can attend. Nevertheless, it is promising that people are increasingly joining the local therapy program rather than more affordable programs.

Studying in North Florida in the US, Khamara-Lani didn't see herself or her culture reflected in the program, instructors, classmates, course material, or the local area—a wealthy white suburb. One day in her occupational therapy program, when learning about culture, her classmates all turned to look at her, one of the few students of color. So she asked them, "What, you don't have your own culture?"

It can be lonely as an international student, and code-switching can be necessary to survive. This is something she was familiar with doing back home, based on the diversity in Trini culture. There were two Caribbean students on her courses, from Jamaica and Antigua. Despite being from different island nations, they helped her feel a sense of belonging, and they would discuss how their learnings might apply back home.

Working in a health profession means working with everyone, regardless of race, gender, sexual orientation, and beliefs. These should be requirements for entering the healthcare profession, like the rest of the standards.

Opelousas, Louisiana, a small, poor town in the US with majority Black residents, is where Khamara-Lani completed one of her internships and later worked. It was here that she picked up skills that translated back home because of similar demographics and colonial history. The rural Medicare patient population was demographically very similar to the users of the public health system back home and shared similarities in lifestyles and jobs, being working class, and having to travel far to access care.

Like much of their education system, healthcare is also free in Trinidad and Tobago. Accustomed to healthcare that is accessible for people whether they can afford it or not, Khamara-Lani doesn't like the US healthcare system. In Trinidad and Tobago, insurance is a bonus. Some people have insurance, yet everyone can access healthcare, unlike in the US. This is something she couldn't wrap her head around—for example, without insurance in the US, an occupational therapy session might cost $300 US dollars or more for an evaluation.

Her scholarship comes from public funds, and she wanted the

local public to benefit from her education and training. Being born and raised in Trinidad and Tobago, she wanted her life's work to improve conditions and saw opportunities for what she could offer back home. Her duty was to return home and help her grandmother and her people. She dedicated herself to working in her country and supporting her family and community, giving up on opportunities for a higher income elsewhere for a higher purpose.

Typically, occupational therapists working in the public sector work in mental health settings. Khamara-Lani is the Head of Occupational Therapy at St. Ann's Hospital, the country's only psychiatric hospital. There are three occupational therapists and six aides in her department, contrasting with the US, where there are significantly fewer and sometimes no aides in a department full of therapists. An outpatient pediatric clinic for children in the public school system has also recently started. This is progressive for the limited scope of government-sponsored services, focused primarily on mental health. Khamara-Lani also works part time in a Florida-based private clinic in Trinidad.

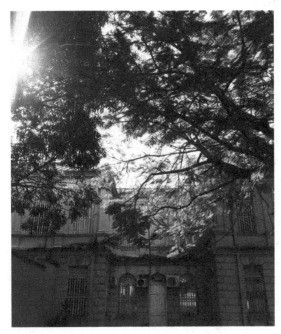

Figure 13.2: Façade of St. Ann's Hospital

Interventions are influenced by nature and culture—for example, the use of coconut trees and local fruits, flying kites, outdoor cooking, and religious integrations are part of activities in the hospital.

Occupation is usually confused with work, so she leans into it. When she explains what occupational therapy is, she starts where people are. She asks people to think of their life as a job. From the time they are born, they have jobs they need to do, and as they grow, some jobs are taken from people supporting them and given to them to do for themselves. "These are jobs that you need in order to do the work of being alive," she sums up. Rather than redefine it, she works with people where they are.

The country's colonial history deeply impacts mental health, resulting in it being a taboo subject. In countries that have been historically oppressed, where the people are seen as less than or sub-human, labels might result in people feeling even more dehumanized. The country has rich and diverse cultures, and in most religions practiced locally, there is a ceremony to try and remove mental illness. Patients often seek spiritual healing first before medical help. It's common for people not to accept the label of their diagnosis.

Othering is also common, where people believe that they can't have a disability or diagnosis, that it happens to other people. Even local music uses lyrics to reinforce this thinking, referring to the psychiatric hospital as a madhouse. The hospital is part of the community but still apart from it. When they find out Khamara-Lani works there, they ask her what it's like on the inside. She tells them to find out if they know someone who has stayed there and ask them. They are usually offended, and she normalizes it because they likely do know someone who is or has been there for care.

In Western countries, acknowledging mental illness and accepting a diagnosis can be empowering. Still, it's critical to recognize who can claim their disability, have it empower them, and see it as part of their identity, and who is further disadvantaged by the label. In some local cultures, making a joke about it is a way to accept and claim identity. The context doesn't always translate, but this is common and shouldn't be judged by someone who hasn't lived it.

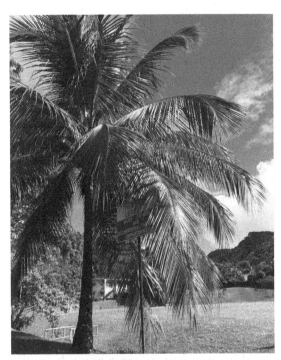

Figure 13.3: Occupational therapy department sign and lush property around St. Ann's Hospital

Mental health is more of a social problem than a medical one—people with mental illness access free medication, mental health clinics, check-ups, and hospital visits. However, there are very limited social placements. So, families only know of the psychiatric hospital as a means of support. Some patients have lived there from their teenage years until the end of life, not necessarily due to unmanaged symptoms. There is inadequate community placement or support for life outside the hospital.

Trinidad and Tobago's healthcare system is modeled after England's because of their colonial ties, despite 60 years of independence. When the British left, self-sustaining social systems weren't put in place for locals. The old frameworks remained, and because foreign is often perceived as better, they keep adapting to fit instead of building new ones for and by the people. There's even a belief that foreign-trained occupational therapists are better than locally trained ones.

Occupational therapy is a helping profession, and we go into this profession with good intentions and consider ourselves good people. Barriers to occupational engagement are systemic. With systemic issues, there is both a personal and a collective responsibility. Khamara-Lani isn't sure what her future path will be, if she is interested in a political position with power and influence or if it will be community-based involvement. She recognizes that our influence has to be on a systemic level to address policies, procedures, and the root of the barriers.

Trinidad and Tobago is rich in cultures from recent immigration and indentured systems of the past, and many languages are spoken throughout the country. English and Trinidad Patois are most commonly spoken, with slightly different dialects in Tobago. Though one nation with more similarities than differences, the islands have varying histories. Tobago has more Dutch and African influences, while Trinidad has more Indian influences and is more culturally diverse.

Khamara-Lani lives in Diego Martin, near the capital of Trinidad, where most services are. The country is split into five regional health authority systems. However, there is only one psychiatric hospital, with psychiatric wards in each health authority. Patients often go to a local general hospital to stabilize before they are transferred to the psychiatric hospital, ferried across islands as needed. Though they can go directly to the psychiatric hospital.

She describes the system as a beehive. Each regional health authority is responsible for all health services in their area. They typically handle acute psychiatric cases and transfer patients to St. Ann's Hospital if they cannot be managed within regional care. People can self-admit, be referred by private physicians, or be brought in from the community by paramedics often accompanied by the police. After discharge from the hospital, they are followed up at their local wellness center for medication and additional care. Mental health officers complete at-home checks as needed. Families often call on the police for help.

In many parts of the world, the problem with police responding to mental health crises is that some people in crisis are harmed or killed by the police. In Trinidad and Tobago, there was a local pilot program training municipal police officers, who often respond with mental health professionals to behavioral health calls in the community or family requests for assistance. All community-level police officers were trained in mental health by staff in the psychiatric hospital, and there is a plan to train all police officers in mental health by 2023, which has not been completed at the time of writing of this book in April 2023. There is also an ongoing relationship between community-level police and mental health officers, who are typically registered nurses with additional training to give medication in the field and do wellness checks. Similar programs have started in some major cities in the US, including removing police altogether from the response.

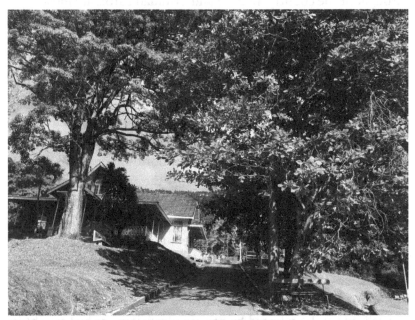

Figure 13.4: Road leading to the occupational therapy building at St. Ann's Hospital. On the left is a poui tree

Occupational therapy in Trinidad and Tobago started in mental health, so there is not much focus on pediatrics or physical rehabilitation in the public sector. Some of these areas are addressed in private practice, but the country is based on a public health system. Therefore, people who can't afford it will not be accessing needed services.

Access to resources and tools is an enormous barrier. Specifically, standardized tests are extremely expensive and don't consider the local population. An assessment that costs $500 USD converted to local currency would be equivalent to almost TT $3500, greater than the monthly minimum wage. Most occupational therapists have to spend their own money to buy what they need.

In the US, Khamara-Lani was used to co-treating and being part of multidisciplinary teams. There was administrative support, software for documentation, filing, and paperwork systems in place—all of which she had to create when returning home to Trinidad and Tobago. Discharges came with plans for home or community outpatient services. There are not as many sub-specialties in Trinidad and Tobago, and therapy roles overlap to cover more services people can benefit from.

Systems and processes are non-existent. Evaluation, intake, and discharge forms aren't available and have to be created. Additional skills are needed beyond clinical, such as managerial, administrative, and organization skills.

There is a belief that anyone can be an occupational therapist. People think Khamara-Lani is a glorified craft teacher. Non-occupational therapists often tell her that they can do what she does. We do "simple things for complicated reasons," she explains. In some cases, aides are used as a replacement for therapists. With the Regulatory Council and Occupational Therapy Board, she is working on addressing this.

The therapist shortage is no longer a major challenge. It's still an issue, but the numbers are growing. Currently, there are 32 occupational therapists in the country. In 2009, there were fewer than ten. There are about ten occupational therapy assistants, and no licensing or regulation for aides or assistants.

The Occupational Therapy and Speech Language Pathology Board created a mentorship program for occupational therapists with less than a year of experience. They are required to be part of a 12-month mentorship program to build community and connection and help transfer textbook knowledge into the local context.

Khamara-Lani's hope for occupational therapy in the country

is to better integrate into the healthcare and education systems. She wants every major healthcare facility to have an occupational therapy department and have the profession expand beyond mental health into all areas of need. This will require the numbers to grow significantly.

Globally, she wants us not to have to explain occupational therapy because people already know what we do. The global occupational therapy community must reflect international practitioners and service users. Cooking outside on a fire should be considered just as civilized as cooking on a stovetop. Culture has to be part of everything we do in practice. There's no one way to be. The basis of what we do is activity analysis. In any activity, there are infinite ways to do it. The differences should be embraced and appreciated.

She lives in the same house she grew up in, which is only 15 minutes away from St. Ann's. The hospital has people from all over the country. She has a diverse background and has been exposed to many cultures and religious traditions. It's hard to be closed-minded with so much diversity around. From colonial history and indentureship to the oil industry, there are people from all over the world living in Trinidad. Tobago has the world's oldest protected rainforest and is a bird watchers' paradise, so it also brings people from all over. There are a lot of cultures present, but you have to be curious about them to find commonality and connection. The complicated and complex cultures of the country have prepared her to work with different people.

Racism is not as problematic as classism. Though racism exists, there isn't the power behind it that there is in majority white countries. A lighter skin tone is often associated with a higher class. As she previously mentioned, to become an occupational therapist, one would have to leave the country to study; so many occupational therapists came from more affluent backgrounds, had international ties, or received scholarships. Now that the profession is easier for locals to access, it has become more representative of the population.

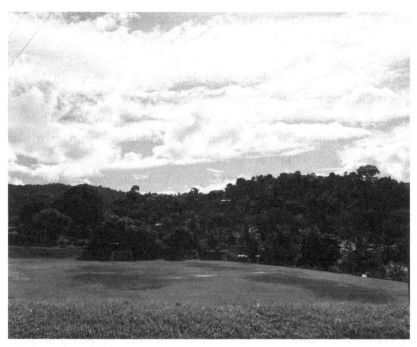

Figure 13.5: Lush hillsides and area surrounding St. Ann's Hospital

She describes the country as "a force of nature" with "a spirit of resistance that runs through the land." Caribbeans are passionate and proud of their heritage. "When you meet a Caribbean person somewhere else, you know they are Caribbean." She describes people in the diaspora generations removed from their island roots carrying a flag of their heritage and talking about their culture. There is energy and a connection to the land, nature, and spirituality. As a culture, so much has been taken from them. They have been told their ways are wrong, demonic, or impure, so they resist by fully appreciating life. Caribbeans do things passionately and enjoy having "a lime," hanging out, and having a good time.

"Live yuh life like yuh playing mas," she shares the lyrics to a song by David Rudder, a Trinidadian calypsonian. Mas is short for masquerade, lively Carnival parade festivities with a masquerade band full of colorful costumes, upbeat live music, and dancing. This invokes a vivid scene as she describes her people as vibrant, enthusiastic, engaged, and speaking loudly and quickly.

"As much as there's a passion and pride and a liveliness about us, there's also a pain that runs very deeply through the country," she says, listing the high incidences of crime, a history of gangs, and drug trade routes. People pretend that colonial history still doesn't affect them, so policies are not challenged. The legacy persists in small ways, like dress codes and obvious political racial divisions. The two major racial categories, Afro-Trinidadian and Indo-Trinidadian, also represent the two main political parties.

Her advice to readers is that we get to know ourselves, who we are, what we want to do, and who we want to be. If she didn't know who she was and what brought her peace, she wouldn't have been able to extend herself into leadership roles. Know ourselves before we give anywhere else. Challenging work can only be sustained by prioritizing self-care and tying professional goals to personal fulfillment.

Now that you have read Khamara-Lani's story, please take some time to think about occupational therapy in your context. Your perspectives are meant to shift the more you learn. So take your time and revisit your earlier responses.

SUGGESTED NEXT STEPS

Reflection: What is the healthcare system like where you live? How does politics impact healthcare? What are common barriers to occupational engagement in your region?

Action: Take Khamara-Lani's advice, and get to know yourself. Journal your responses to the following: Who are you? What do you want to do? Who do you want to be?

CHAPTER 14

BANGLADESH: Razia Sultana

It's Saturday morning in Dhaka, and Razia calls in from her husband's office. They are both off work today, and she travels there to ensure that the connection is solid and we can speak without interruptions. Unfortunately, internet service can be problematic in Bangladesh, and her video feed is delayed. I see her briefly before she turns the camera off to improve connectivity. She has straight black hair tied back and is wearing a black and white checkered salwar with a red orna, a long scarf.

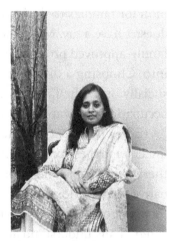

Figure 14.1: Razia sitting down wearing a salwar kameez

Razia Sultana is a Muslim woman and mental health occupational therapist in the capital city of Dhaka. An occupational therapist of eight years, she was the country's first to work in mental health. Most occupational therapists work in physical rehabilitation settings for the Centre for the Rehabilitation of the Paralysed (CRP), an NGO.

Though the first Bangladeshi occupational therapy graduates in the country completed their studies in 1976, it wasn't until 2000 that World Federation of Occupational Therapists accredited the program in Bangladesh. That first program closed, then in 1996 a diploma course started. Following that, in 1999, a bachelor's program opened at the Bangladesh Health Professions Institute, an academic institute of CRP affiliated with Dhaka University. Currently, there is an occupational therapy assistant program and bachelor's degree course, which includes four years of studies with one year of internships. A master's program will start at the end of the year.

Having never heard of occupational therapy, Razia wanted to be a doctor but didn't make the competitive program. Hoping to work in healthcare, she went to CRP to learn about her options after a relative told her about their work. CRP has physical, occupational, and speech therapy training programs. Without knowing much about it, she decided on occupational therapy because a friend had chosen it.

Starting the program was controversial. In Bangladesh, it's common for families to decide the course of studies, while the student doesn't have a say. Medicine and engineering are the most popular, family-approved professions, which makes them even harder to get into. Choosing a different career or subject is often not accepted socially or by the family. Additionally, when she decided to study occupational therapy, it was relatively unknown.

In her first year of studies, she was frustrated. Struggling to understand the profession herself, it was hard to explain occupational therapy to people and even more difficult to explain in Bangla, her native tongue. Most people thought she was studying to be a physical therapist or doctor. However, once she completed her studies, she could finally understand and explain the profession.

There are no Bangla textbooks. Textbooks in programs come from Western countries. Teachers must adapt the information to the language, culture, and context. For example, bathing and toileting look very different in Bangladesh than in Europe or North America, and eating food with hands rather than utensils is more common. Assessment forms are not available in Bangla either. There is no way to maintain standardized assessments when these are informally translated. Some things don't make sense or translate culturally.

In her fourth year, she began internship placements. No occupational therapist was working in mental health settings until Karen Heaslip came to volunteer from the UK. Razia met with her, and they worked together to find a way to start mental health occupational therapy in Bangladesh. Razia was the first student to complete an internship in a mental health hospital. They set up the program so new students would rotate every three months to provide full-time, year-round coverage of occupational therapy services with student therapists.

Karen raised funds and helped create a position for an occupational therapist in a mental health hospital. The job was through CRP, and the salary was to be paid through the donations Karen raised. Once Razia passed her internships, she was interviewed and got the position to work at the National Institute of Mental Health and Hospital in Dhaka, becoming the first mental health occupational therapist in Bangladesh.

Before her current role at SAJIDA Foundation, a non-profit NGO, she worked for CRP in a community mental health day center. SAJIDA's team visited various mental health organizations, including the day center, to grow their mental health program. As a result, they recruited her to work with them as Deputy Program Manager and the only occupational therapist in the organization. Excited to make a more significant impact, she took on the role and hopes it will make room for more occupational therapists working in community mental health.

SAJIDA has a residential mental health rehabilitation facility, provides tele-mental health counseling, Bangladesh's first emotional support and suicide prevention helpline, and a diploma mental health training program, and is building supportive housing communities. Razia is responsible for the supported housing and residential facility. This housing program is based on an Indian model from The Banyan, providing clinical and social-based comprehensive mental health services.

SAJIDA's mental health team went to visit The Banyan's program. Inspired by its success in providing comprehensive mental healthcare in a community setting, they are replicating it in Bangladesh. The plan is to provide housing and services to low-income and ultra-poor people with severe mental illness whose families cannot or do not want to support them or who don't want to go back to live with their families. Initially, SAJIDA is renting a house to create a family environment with four to five people living in one flat. Within the house, there will be a staff member supporting residents and a case manager or care coordinator. Razia will supervise the team.

Once again, she is representing many firsts. She is the first occupational therapist with SAJIDA working on the first supported housing facility in Bangladesh. She acknowledges that she is breaking barriers, but at the same time, navigating unknown spaces is taxing. Many of her occupational therapy colleagues, not in mental health, don't understand what she does. And no one in the country is doing anything similar for her to learn from and problem solve with.

The government does not officially recognize occupational therapy; therefore, there are no licensing or regulatory standards. It's been a few years since the Bangladesh Occupational Therapy Association submitted paperwork for the government to consider occupational therapy in Bangladesh and open government positions. Without these standards, anyone without a degree or training can apply to be an occupational therapist within the limited government hospital positions. The lack of requirement for appropriate training diminishes what occupational therapy can offer, does not benefit those receiving care, and is demotivating for people with a bachelor's degree and formal training in applying for these positions.

Many Bangladesh-trained occupational therapists leave the country for better work opportunities and pay. Currently, there are 363 occupational therapists qualified in Bangladesh, with 37 living and working abroad. Razia feels connected to her work in Bangladesh. Her family has asked her to consider working abroad to grow professionally, but she would rather stay in her home country and grow the profession. The hope is that her new role will allow her to realize this goal.

Occupation in Bangla is টেশা (*pesha*), which translates to work. Therapists don't use this term, instead sticking to occupation and occupational therapy in English, even though they work with clients in Bangla. Bangla is most commonly spoken as it is their schooling medium. English is more commonly used in higher education, so it is not accessible to everyone.

The population Razia works with is mostly from Dhaka, with some coming from further cities like Sylhet for work or family. Most are illiterate, having limited educational opportunities, so a relatable explanation of occupational therapy works best.

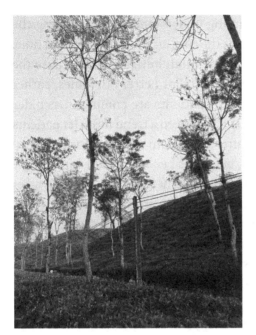

Figure 14.2: Tea garden in Sylhet

The continuation of services is problematic. The cultural significance of independence isn't valued by families that are used to helping each other. Poor patients are more likely to rely on family support, so independence isn't their most important goal, further deprioritizing occupational therapy.

Services are expensive, so they aren't eager to continue, hoping for a quick and easy solution like taking medication, or a short hospital stay. Occupational therapy services take time to show progress and are only available in large cities, making them difficult to access.

People outside the city have to travel to Dhaka. They are more likely to see the value in visiting a doctor, which can cost anywhere from 500 to 1000 taka for a single visit, usually once a month or less. However, occupational therapy is something they don't understand and is typically preventative or rehabilitative. Occupational therapy sessions are about 400 taka—more than the daily minimum wage—and require multiple sessions a week for a service they might not even understand, so they are less likely to spend time and money on these services.

Many barriers exist, including understanding and valuing the benefits of occupational therapy, the cost, access, priorities, and time. In the case of children, services are often initiated late because the mother is at home helping the child. For better outcomes, earlier intervention is critical, but many patients are coming in as older children, often pre-teens. Razia has noticed a trend for older patients coming in three or four years after an incident or injury. Family members have been helping them, but it has become a hardship, so they want to pursue therapy to gain independence. By then, progress takes longer, and the benefit is not as great because interventions haven't been implemented early enough.

With mental health, there is even more stigma. Acceptance of diagnosis and medication is also problematic. Either people don't want to take medication, or their families can't afford long-term use. People who are hesitant to receive medical care are even warier about counseling and occupational therapy services.

Referrals to occupational therapy services are another hurdle. For physical rehabilitation, some doctors will assign a home exercise program, and, believing they are covering all needed services, will therefore not refer patients to physical or occupational therapy. If the government recognized the profession, services would be more accessible and affordable and eventually better understood. When Razia worked in the government hospital, services were free. Therefore, more people would access, accept, and continue care as recommended.

The multidisciplinary team approach is not common in Bangladesh. Razia tries to connect with other professionals and build multidisciplinary teams with psychologists, psychiatrists, social workers, and nurses. She did this at the day center and plans to continue it in her new role.

Bangladesh has no public or government-based health insurance, though some people have private insurance. There are private hospitals with better care, but the services are too expensive for the average person to access. Government hospitals offer free or inexpensive services. However, their staffing is too low to meet the needs of everyone who needs care. NGOs like CRP are trying to fill these gaps, but they are donation-based, making sustainability a concern and availability limited throughout the country.

In a recent development, occupational therapists have begun to work in schools. Some prominent Bangladeshi figures have become autism advocates, bringing awareness into politics and social life. As a result, people are becoming more aware of autism and accepting related services.

Razia's voice lightens and gains some energy; she loves working in mental health and connecting with clients. Helping people meet their goals is fulfilling for her. At the day center, the basis of occupational therapy services is group activities, which are meaningful and enjoyable to the clients and a way to learn more about them. Positive caregiver and family feedback for clients showing progress at home encourages her to teach more professionals about her work to grow the number of mental health occupational therapists in the country.

As the first and only mental health occupational therapist, she found it challenging to establish her role and place in the profession. Occupational therapy is difficult enough for people to understand, but a role in mental health is even more unique and harder to grasp. There was no one locally that she could have a face-to-face conversation with. Even with more mental health occupational therapists in the country, she is the most experienced, so she has to seek support outside the country.

It has taken time, but Razia finally feels she has enough experience and a network to learn from and problem solve with. She is also a mentor for newer colleagues and helps young professionals experiencing an identity crisis like she did when she was new in her career.

Dhaka is busy and overpopulated. As the capital city, most services are available here, including the most modern medical care. Traffic is a big problem and a lot of time is spent stuck in a vehicle.

Economic conditions are better in Dhaka than in other parts of the country, and things are more modern, but the cost of living is high. Occupational patterns and interests have shifted. People spend more time eating out, which wasn't common until recently. She believes that social media has significantly influenced people to go out and travel more. Internet access is available nationwide, so this is a national trend. People are less engaged with each other and more involved in social media, a significant change for a community-oriented culture.

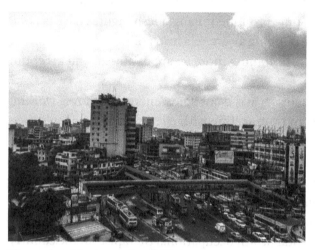

Figure 14.3: The busy city of Dhaka

In Bangladeshi culture, like many Asian cultures, parents don't involve their children in chores and household activities. Instead, they want children to focus on school and studies and limit other responsibilities and social activities. Parents or domestic laborers (more common in middle-class and wealthier households) manage household tasks instead of having their children involved. People in homes with domestic workers have someone to shop, cook, drive, clean, wash, and do the majority of instrumental activities of daily living for them.

Some occupational therapists do not participate in these activities for the same reason. This poses a challenge in adapting and teaching others how to engage in them. Razia values having meaningful activities in her life so that she can help others find their own.

Volunteering is not popular in Bangladesh due to overwhelming academic and family pressure. Extracurricular activities are a low priority. When she works with clients, Razia encourages physical activities and hobbies to promote meaningful occupations. Unfortunately, many are not interested in exploring these options. There is a big focus on paid work and earning money, which makes volunteer positions tough to promote, and because volunteering is not encouraged, there aren't many opportunities. Vocational opportunities for people with mental illness and other disabilities are rare. Jobs are very competitive and require high education and skill levels, so people without opportunities to succeed in school and work can't find supportive employment opportunities. There is also a false belief that mentally ill and disabled people should not or cannot work.

Workplaces don't have opportunities for people who have been out of the workforce, and many families discourage their children from participating because they don't think they will succeed. The lack of support and opportunity is compounded by the lack of value placed on individual interests. If one isn't in school and cannot get a job, then few options remain. It's challenging to motivate people to engage in and find interests or try things that would benefit them outside monetary gain. The traffic problem, often taking double the expected time to reach a destination, makes it harder to get people involved in activities in the community.

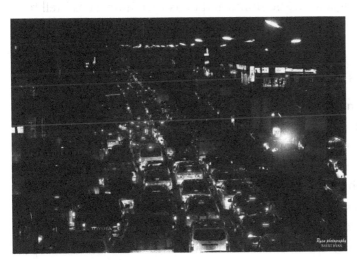

Figure 14.4: Dhaka night traffic

Income inequality is stark and only growing, increasing the need for medical care, while making access to care less possible. Part-time jobs are rare, which is problematic for working mothers and people who can't work full-time. This affects occupational therapists as well, as there are no part-time positions. It's difficult to find a job after a gap in employment, especially for mothers who have stayed at home to raise young children. There is a lack of day care facilities, so they have no choice but to stay at home. Razia hopes part-time positions will be available on her team as it grows.

Her dream is to create supported employment or job coaching programs in Bangladesh. There are vocational training programs in the country; however, it is a challenge to find jobs that are willing to provide support. When people find work, they often don't last long because of the lack of support at work and bullying from co-workers.

Globally, Razia wants more collaboration. While she has benefitted from networking internationally, she hopes that this can become better established. She doesn't feel as connected with occupational therapists in her own country, so she has connected with an occupational therapist abroad to discuss practice concerns and treatment ideas, leaving her more confident and encouraged.

Razia turns her camera back on to say goodbye and invite me to visit Bangladesh. She smiles and nods with interest as I tell her I would love to come and visit my ancestral home someday.

SUGGESTED NEXT STEPS

Reflection: What are the occupational therapy specialties in your region? Are there any misunderstood areas of practice? Why do you think this is, and how can it be remedied?

Action: What areas of practice are you inexperienced in? Look up referral sources for the most commonly requested or needed areas to refer clients you cannot best serve. If it's an area you are interested in learning about, find a book or course to learn more.

CHAPTER 15

HAITI: Ramona Joëlle Adrien

Ramona Joëlle Adrien is a Haitian occupational therapist now studying in Canada. With only a year and a half of practical experience, she teaches and supports students in the Haitian occupational therapy program. An Evangelical, she is in the process of publishing a worship song and writing a book. Passionate about everything she does, Ramona speaks with her words, body, and hands. Powerful and petite, she has long black braids pulled back with burgundy oval glasses and a bright yellow sweatshirt, while sitting in a shared apartment with roommates near her university.

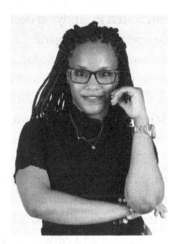

Figure 15.1: Close-up photo of Ramona

After the catastrophic earthquake in 2010, the number of disabled people skyrocketed in Haiti, and there weren't enough healthcare providers or facilities to help. People lost limbs, jobs, function, and mobility. Her mother is a physician, and in 2012 as a high school student, Ramona volunteered at the hospital where her mom worked. A team of occupational and physical therapy students from the Université de Sherbrooke in Canada, where she is currently studying, came to complete their internship. She translated French into Creole during the therapy sessions for the visiting students who didn't speak the local language. There, she fell in love with occupational therapy and knew it was what she wanted to do.

After graduation, she wanted to join that Canadian occupational therapy program. However, it was closed to international students. Instead, she went to business school at home and then got an opportunity to study pre-physical therapy in the US. It would have been a good opportunity to later pursue a master's or doctorate in occupational therapy.

She had to return home because of family issues before completing the program. Coincidentally, the person facilitating the student therapist program contacted Ramona's mother and asked if Ramona was interested in studying occupational therapy. A local program would be opening in Léogâne (Leyogàn in Haitian Creole) at the Université Épiscopale d'Haïti. So far, it has graduated two cohorts of students in occupational therapy and three in physical therapy from the Faculté des Sciences de Réhabilitation de Léogâne, the Department of the Sciences of Rehabilitation of Léogâne. Léogâne is about 45 minutes from the capital of Port-au-Prince, where Ramona is from.

This four-and-a-half-year bachelor's program was developed by the Haiti Rehabilitation Foundation, a non-profit working to make rehabilitation sustainable in Haiti. They are partnered with Université de Sherbrooke and additional universities and faculties abroad for support and educational materials.

Ramona graduated with seven physical and two other occupational therapists in the first cohort. She is one of the first three Haitian occupational therapists to be trained in the country. After completing her internships, she worked at Respire Haiti, an organization in Gressier, 15 minutes north of the occupational therapy school in Léogâne. Respire Haiti's mission is "to encourage, educate and empower restavèks, orphans and vulnerable children." And their vision is "a Haiti in which all children have access to safe community, education and equal opportunity." Restavèks are child slaves or domestic servants. They are less likely to attend school and more likely to experience emotional, physical, and sexual abuse. In 2012, over 300,000, possibly 500,000, children in Haiti were living as restavèks, given up by their parents, who couldn't afford to raise them, hoping they would have a chance for a better life (Gilbert *et al.*, 2018).

Respire Haiti has a school, clinic, and community program. They organize parent support groups as well. Ramona completed her internship here and later worked for a year and a half before suddenly quitting. She worked in the clinic and school special education program. Although she primarily worked with children, adults in the program needed therapy too. There are not enough occupational therapists in the country to have specializations. They are generalists working with all populations. Respire has a home program, but it has been on hold with the COVID-19 pandemic and socio-political conflicts.

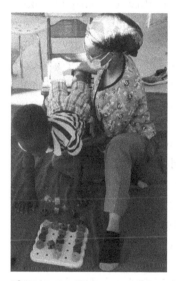

Figure 15.2: Ramona working with a child

Ramona's clinical experience was cut short because of political instability and violence. She had to quit her job without any notice or warning. A year later, she still hasn't got over it. Sharing a map on the screen, she goes over what has been happening over the past two years. There are three main roadways in the country branching out from the capital. She would use Route Nationale 2 to go from her home in Port-au-Prince to her work further south in Gressier. At the border, gangs took over the area. There is really only one way through. A second road exists but it was even less safe.

In the summer of 2021, Haiti's President Jovenel Moïse was assassinated, accelerating the already existing gang violence. By December 2021, Ramona was exposed to more of this violence on her weekly route to and from work. Sometimes, roadblocks stranded her on the road with other drivers, bullets flying across the roadway while gangs fought each other—civilians caught in the crossfire on their way to work and school. This escalated further when the gangs attacked the local police. Two officers were killed and their bodies never returned. People using the route were now at risk of being kidnapped. Ramona worked for another couple of months, thanking God for keeping her safe, but as the route became more dangerous, she could no longer take the risk.

These barriers to survival are a daily reality for many Haitians. Gang violence is only worsening, preventing many Haitians from leaving their homes to work, go to school, seek necessary medical care, and access food and basic necessities. This is making people even more vulnerable to illnesses like cholera. Recent cholera outbreaks have hit locals hard, amid an already unthinkable humanitarian crisis (World Health Organization, 2022).

Almost 90 percent of the population does not have access to drinking water in their homes (World Bank, 2020). Most water sources are contaminated because of poor sanitation systems. Only a third of the population has access to basic sanitation. The majority of diseases in the country are waterborne, putting infants and children at the greatest risk. Electricity is not always available, and people have to walk miles to access water and food.

Most therapy services are provided by NGOs funded by donations. They offer services at a low price. There is also insurance that can cover therapy services. Without these options, services are unaffordable and inaccessible. Where Ramona worked, services were offered at a monthly fee of 350 gourdes, more than some people make in a day. In some cities, it could cost double that for one session. Costs vary depending on the location and organization.

Occupational therapy is not recognized by the government. The practice is not regulated and because of political and social turmoil, it is a bigger challenge to realize. Without government approval, it can't be part of the standard covered healthcare services.

Locals who go abroad to study don't return to Haiti to practice. Association Haïtienne D'Ergothérapeutes (Haitian Association of Occupational Therapy) tracks occupational therapists in the country. When Ramona became an occupational therapist, only one occupational therapist was Haitian, and he is both a physical and occupational therapist. The President of the Association is Haitian but lives and works in the US. The three who graduated in the first cohort, including Ramona, were the first local practicing occupational therapists. The remaining therapists have come from abroad but have lived in the country for a long time, so they understand the context. They are invested in the country because it is their home too.

This is in contrast to foreign providers coming in and telling people what to do without intimately understanding Haitian life, which often happens in a country with limited resources in need of rehabilitation services. Saviorism and short-term medical missions, including those conducted by occupational therapists, are not new to Haiti and can cause more harm than good (Schlegel & Mathieson, 2020). These stints don't address structural problems and can cause an overreliance on outside support rather than bolstering what existing communities are doing. The positive impacts are even less notable without an understanding of the culture.

With Ramona in Canada, there are now five occupational therapists who live in Haiti: two who graduated with her, one who happens to be both an occupational and physical therapist, two who practice there but live abroad sometimes, and one currently on leave. The next cohort will graduate with five students at the end of this year. That will bring the number of practicing occupational therapists in the country up to ten.

With prior experience studying abroad and now officially in a master's program, Ramona was always planning to return to Haiti. Her vision has consistently been clear: "Neither the US nor Canada needs me." Her people have been through a lot, historically, politically, economically, and with natural disasters. Haiti was the first Black-led republic, fighting to free themselves from French enslavers in 1791, but indebted to them in exchange for freedom until 1947 (Porter *et al.*, 2022). Generations of Haitians paid off descendants of enslavers, making France even wealthier and leaving Haiti the poorest country in the Western Hemisphere.

Because of much instability and uncertainty, people are constantly made to change their occupations, roles, and ways of living. It causes psychological, physiological, and physical stress and uncertainty. But, in the process, they relearn to exist, be, and do. This is why occupational therapy is so appealing to Ramona, supporting people in just being.

She is determined to help her people live better, easier, and fuller lives. Growing up, she saw children cast aside because they were different. The grading system in schools requires a limited threshold for passing students. In most schools, if a student doesn't pass with 65 percent (50 percent in some schools) in classes like math or physics, they are retained and have to repeat. This can be repeated over and over. Ramona was drawn to school interventions to change the punitive system, help students succeed, and have parents, teachers, and administrators realize that students can achieve more with support.

For everyone in the country to receive access to basic care, Ramona must be at home. She can't do this work abroad. With a sense of duty to her people, she has a personal responsibility to ensure that painful and deadly situations improve. If everyone leaves for an education and better opportunities, who is left behind to fight for the people who remain?

After completing her master's degree at the Université de Sherbrooke in Quebec, Canada, Ramona plans to open a facility in Haiti with multiple services, including physical, occupational, and speech therapies and psychology. She will be the first Haitian-trained local occupational therapist with a master's degree. There are not enough Haitian teachers in the local program. If occupational therapy is to be a profession in Haiti for Haitians, then they should be taught by a Haitian occupational therapist.

Haitian Creole is spoken throughout the country and is most commonly used in practice. French is taught in school and is the second most common language. English is introduced from first grade to high school, and some students can read in English and communicate with simple greetings. Use of this language is not common, and without practice, the language is difficult to maintain.

Ramona is fluent because she was sent to live with family in the US after the earthquake.

Okipasyon is occupation in Haitian Creole. The profession is *terapi okipasyonèl* or *terapi fonksyonèl*, functional therapy. Ramona's explanation is simple: she tells people she is there to help them do what they have or want to do every day.

The structural and systemic barriers are significant. Occupational therapy is not recognized by the government, a political problem. Everything in Haiti is political. This turmoil is embedded in their culture.

Ramona is currently worried sick about her family back home, as there have been riots in the streets every day for the past seven days. A few days ago, her mom woke up to no drinking water in the house. This uncertainty impacts schools, healthcare, and everything in life. For example, there is no access to materials for making splints. They are too expensive and not available in the country. Even if there were funds to pay for the material and shipping, the ports are blocked, so there is no way to get them.

The whole day could be spent explaining barriers to me. There are also cultural challenges. Vodou is commonly practiced in Haiti. There's a familiar belief that when someone is ill or disabled, they are cursed and did something wrong to deserve it. It's challenging for some people to understand that there is a medical explanation, and it is not their fault. So, Ramona would work with parents to help them understand that there was no curse on their child, there was an explanation, and with therapy, their function could improve. The parent support group helped debunk these myths without directly confronting long-held traditional beliefs.

Ramona is used to translating everything she has learned professionally from non-Haitian teachers into the Haitian context, specifically translating what is meant for white people into a context for Black Haitians. Typical therapy materials are not available. There is little to no access to things like string, beads, and putty to work on fine motor skills.

Standardized tests and measures for leisure, productivity, and self-care are not always relevant. For instance, most people don't go out to restaurants to eat in Haiti unless they are wealthy. Street restaurants, comparable to food trucks, are popular and more accessible. Few children know how to play with puzzles because they don't have access to them. Outdoor activities like climbing trees, playing in rivers, and barefoot exploration are more common. As the profession grows in the country, it's critical to have assessments, evaluations, and interventions that fit the local context and culture.

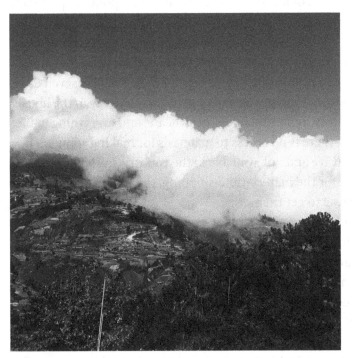

Figure 15.3: Lush hillsides and landscape in Port-au-Prince

Assessments normed on people with access to running water, electricity, infrastructure, social systems, and resources can be a waste of time and money when these contexts do not apply. Often this can look like people having more deficits when they can actually function well in their own environments and contexts. With the shift to Haitian occupational therapists teaching and working locally, the Haitian context can one day be part of textbooks, assessments, and interventions. The local program is working toward this.

I ask Ramona to describe Haiti, and I make the mistake of

mentioning resilience. I meant to say resistance, though resilience is commonly used to describe surviving difficult situations outside one's control. Instead of celebrating resilience, we should be working to change systems that force people to be resilient to survive.

She doesn't want to discuss resilience. Haiti is full of natural resources, which is why it falls "prey to predators," she explains, "Haitians do not have any choice but to be resilient."

There is a strong sense of family in Haiti. Wherever you go, you are family. This is one of the greatest assets in doing community or family interventions. Haitian families are typically always together. It's rare for someone to come to therapy alone. Even if they don't have relatives available, someone in the neighborhood will bring them in for sessions, take them to appointments, and provide help when they need it. Haiti has been tested at many points in history, but the people remain unified. "We've got each other's back," she exclaims with pride.

There's a push for independence in occupational therapy, but that's not always a goal here. Community support is accepted and given, a beautiful thing.

It's difficult to advocate for the profession and services because the numbers are so few. Currently, the mental health and social aspects of occupational therapy are not systematically embedded despite, in recent years, clinical supervisors raising awareness of the importance of addressing these areas in practice and students implementing learnings well. Only physical disabilities are associated with occupational therapy and other rehabilitation services. Therapists are not working in psychiatric settings yet.

Ramona wants occupational therapy to become a well-known profession in the country and officially recognized so that anyone can benefit and access care. Globally, she wants inclusion to be realized with testing, evaluations, and interventions contextualized for all people and cultures.

Her advice to readers is to be open-minded and ready to learn. We should be adaptable as professionals and open to various cultures.

The limited resources in Haiti impact the availability of teachers on campus, so everything is done online. Ramona puts a call out to anyone interested in teaching in the program in Haiti, including guest lecturers.

We are both eager for her to return home and put the knowledge she brings back into action. More local students will see themselves succeeding when she becomes a professor because of her representation. It's wonderful that people with resources and privilege come from the outside and bring support, but there are limitations in how locals respond to them. The limitations are essential to acknowledge. Trust and connection are more automatic with someone local, and when services are sustainable; therefore, investing in and supporting local clinicians should be prioritized over voluntourism.

SUGGESTED NEXT STEPS

Reflection: What is your country's political, social, and cultural history? Try finding the people's history, and if applicable, that of any people colonized or forced onto the land. What misconceptions did you have about developing countries and medical missions to benefit disabled people? What have you learned that can help you understand how to better approach people from different cultures?

Action: Reach out to a program in another country and offer to guest lecture or partner/mentor with a student or clinician. If you don't have any known contacts, email DisruptOT at disruptotsummit@ gmail.com to connect with our partnership program or programs looking for guest speakers.

References

Gilbert, L., Reza. A., Mercy. J.A., Lea, V., *et al.* (2018). "The experience of violence against children in domestic servitude in Haiti: Results from the Violence Against Children Survey, Haiti 2012." *Child Abuse & Neglect*, 76: 184–193.

Porter, C., Méheut, C., Apuzzo, M., & Gebrekidan, S. (2022, May 20). "The Root of Haiti's Misery: Reparations to Enslavers." *The New York Times*. www.nytimes. com/2022/05/20/world/americas/haiti-history-colonized-france.html.

Schlegel, S.M. & Mathieson, K. (2020). "Occupational therapy in Haiti: A pilot study to identify intervention methods used during short-term medical missions." *Occupational Therapy International*, 2020, 4198402, https://doi.org/10.1155/2020/4198402.

World Bank. (2020). *As Haiti Braces for the COVID-19 Pandemic, Water, Sanitation, and Hygiene Are More Important Than Ever*. www.worldbank.org/en/news/feature/2020/05/29/as-haiti-braces-for-the-covid-19-pandemic-water-sanitation-and-hygiene-are-more-important-than-ever.

World Health Organization. (2022). *Cholera—Haiti*. www.who.int/emergencies/disease-outbreak-news/item/2022-DON427.

CHAPTER 16

INDIA: Sakshi Tickoo

Sakshi Tickoo introduces herself as a queer, cis femme (woman). From the flat she shares with her mother in Mumbai, Sakshi calls in with a deep blue wall prominently behind her. Her long black hair is pulled back, and she's wearing a gray t-shirt and large black over-ear headphones. A Hindu, born and raised in Mumbai, India, from the Kashmiri Pandit caste, she has been taking time to understand her culture better.

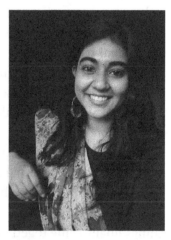

Figure 16.1: Close-up photo of Sakshi

Sakshi has always been fascinated with the body and, as a young child, wanted to be a gynecologist. She would carry a toy medical kit with her everywhere, knowing precisely what she wanted to do from a young age. As she got older, her chronic illnesses impacted her energy levels and she realized that medicine would not be a reality, but that didn't defeat her. An allied health profession would be a good alternative, allowing her to help people while working with the human body.

In India, selecting your profession or institution of study is not an option. A competitive exam throughout the country decides one's course and place of study. Sakshi and her father googled occupational therapy the day she received her results. Neither she nor her father, an astrophysicist, understood what an occupational therapist was, but she was open to the challenge of doing something different.

King Edward Memorial Hospital in Mumbai has the oldest occupational therapy program in Asia, which started in 1950, and was where Sakshi completed her bachelor's studies. The program consists of four years of coursework and six months of internships. There is also an option for a master's degree. Textbooks are primarily from Western countries and are dated. India was colonized by the British, yet the country remains richly diverse in Indian cultures and languages. Moreover, these Western theories do not fit into Indian cultural contexts. For example, textbooks discuss splinting, work hardening (a program to help injured workers return to work), and vocational rehabilitation. Because of costs and barriers to access, these cannot be used or implemented throughout India.

Sakshi found the coursework interesting as it started with anatomy, but things didn't make sense after that. While in school, she was diagnosed with depression and other health problems. Her growing health issues and not understanding the content became a struggle. Unlike Western universities, there is no student support or accommodation for disabilities to help students navigate school and clinical expectations while experiencing health challenges. However, things finally came together in the fourth year, and Sakshi began to connect with occupational therapy. While working with clients, what she learned made more sense, and she was invested in growing in the profession. Treatment plans and internship experiences brought all she learned in the program into something she could understand and appreciate.

Her first placement was in plastic surgery, which pushed her to think beyond the rote range of motion exercises. Without much support, she had to figure out interventions and use of adaptive equipment around the patients' daily occupations. She shares a case where she worked with a Hindu pandit (priest) with a burn injury who wanted to be able to hold *kalash* (a copper vessel essential to Hindu rituals) while performing *hawan* (a ritual in which offerings are made to the fire). The challenge was that any plastic-based materials, like thermoplastic for splints, could not be used during these religious occupations. After hours of brainstorming, using a cuffed cloth and Velcro aid allowed the pandit to perform his work and was a cost-effective solution.

In India, student occupational therapists are left to devise treatment plans and provide care independently rather than training closely under an experienced therapist. She was working on medical floors and seeing patients on her own. It was challenging to provide quality care with ratios of 100 patients to every student therapist, but she took this responsibility seriously. Enjoying the work and getting to know people, she kept notes on everything she learned from each patient to review and continue learning.

In her first job as a school-based occupational therapist, she worked with children from five to 18 years of age. With parental consent, she facilitated groups and worked individually with children with various diagnoses on issues like dressing, toileting, personal hygiene, consent, boundaries, identifying emotions, menstruation, and learning anatomical words for body parts. In her experience, the parents did not agree with her teaching about same-sex relationships, but they were open to more than she expected. Individual sessions focused on skills, while groups emphasized emotional learning. By removing the sexual part from sexuality education, she had a deeper understanding of bringing this material to children.

Sexuality and intimacy are taboo topics in Indian culture, contributing to problems in communicating needs, wants, and if something is wrong. In addition, guilt, shame, and fear dictate actions and choices, adding additional barriers to awareness and openness to learning about these areas of life.

Practicing occupational therapy for three years, Sakshi has already written a book and has a private practice. Her book, *SexCare: A Self-Help Guide to Sexual Wellness*, makes sexuality and pleasure more accessible through a workbook-style guide with activities and sensory strategies.

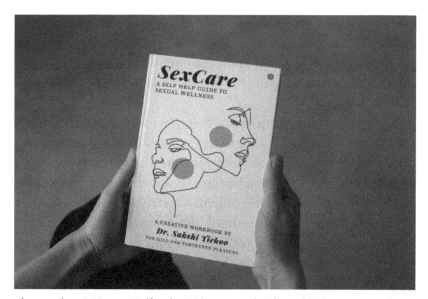

Figure 16.2: *SexCare: A Self-Help Guide to Sexual Wellness* book cover

Seeking to make healthcare more comprehensive, inclusive, and accessible, she set up her telehealth practice, Sex, Love, and OT, where she offers occupational therapy and counseling on sexuality, relationships, and mental health. Website and social media content are designed to offer resources for anyone to learn from and improve, even if they don't work with her. Though Sakshi is based in India, she sees clients worldwide and of all ages via telehealth. So far, the range she's seen is from three to 95. Anything related to sexuality is addressed, from sexual expression, mobility, posture, communication, and boundaries to mental health. She also works with parents, caregivers, and sex workers. Parents and caregivers have children and partners who are disabled and don't have adequate resources to discuss sexuality and sexual expression. Some of the sex workers have disabled clients for whom she helps modify and adapt positions. She also mentors and consults with healthcare professionals wanting to learn more about integrating sexuality into practice, and offers support with complex cases.

A common example of her services is working with women over 35 who want to feel or provide pleasure again. Many married women in heterosexual relationships are made to feel that after a certain age, they cannot feel pleasure or satisfy their partners. Usually, this is more than an issue of desire. It includes family responsibilities, work–life balance, environment, relational support, sensory processing, and physical, physiological, and emotional health. She realizes that it's usually less about sex and more about how other occupational roles affect their occupation of sexuality. So, she works with them to find balance, adapt, and improve all of these areas of life.

Preparing to leave India for Australia, Sakshi will be pursuing a master's in sexology next year. Unfortunately, there aren't many options in India, especially for an occupational therapist, to further her education in sexuality.

India has over 100 major languages. Sakshi uses English, Hindi, Marathi, and Kashmiri in practice. In Hindi, one of India's official languages, occupational therapy is व्यावसायिक चिकित्सा, *vyaavasaayik chikitsa*. She explains to people she works with that occupational therapy includes sex, self-expression, pleasure, and, of course, the more common daily occupations we learn about. Independence is not a focus, as communal culture is prioritized in India. Multi-generational households and living at home in adulthood are typical in India. Her services are not just client-centered. The entire relational unit is part of care because their community and society impact them. She works with individuals, couples, polyamorous relationships, families, and parents.

Surprisingly, she works with more people from smaller cities than in the metropolitan Mumbai area. She has found that they are more open to addressing sexuality than the dense urban population. However, because of the virtual nature of her business and the cost, rural people aren't able to access services.

The biggest challenge she deals with is the taboo of discussing mental health and other Indian cultural norms that prevent people from talking about sex. Sexual scripts, narratives dictated by society and culture, are powerful and Indian culture has a strong, embedded sense of guilt and shame. Often people are worried about their family being upset with them and what other people will think if they find out the person is seeking support for mental health or their sexuality. Many Indian children have high-functioning anxiety because they constantly worry about validation from their parents and those around them. This impacts their sexual worth and roles. She seeks to redefine sex from simply being about pleasure to including joy and intimacy, not just orgasms.

Her clients' journeys bring her the most joy. She empowers them to become and do whatever they want, offering them freedom from the guilt and shame of being free in their bodies and who they are.

Soon after starting her first job and discovering sexuality interventions with children, she got into social media and content creation. In school, she only learned about working with adults with disabilities and illnesses. She never thought working with children in these areas would be meaningful and necessary. So, she took to social media to learn and share her thoughts in a space open and accessible to students and professionals. Since then, she has connected with sexual wellness brands and magazines to talk about sexuality from an occupational therapy perspective, something lacking in mainstream media and occupational therapy education and training.

Because of taboos around sexuality and the culture of guilt and shame, Sakshi is called a pervert and sexually harassed regularly. For this reason, the target audience for online content isn't Indians. Instead, she wants to reach occupational therapists who have no idea where to start when addressing sexuality, and encourage them to include sexuality in assessments, and provide anatomy lessons. Over time, she has started to address the general public, recognizing that many more people can benefit. Though her primary clinical clients are in India, she reaches people worldwide with her content.

She has prepared herself for the nastiness online, being called names and sent graphic sexual images, but there are legitimate safety risks. She is most often harassed by men, and her fear of backlash and cultural policing is warranted. India is a patriarchal country, not unfamiliar with violence against women. There is a real risk of being raped, killed, and her family threatened because she is a young woman discussing forbidden subjects publicly in a conservative country. People think that she is encouraging sex when actually she encourages people to be themselves, live a healthy life, and access information. Ironically, her culture teaches about sex from the

Vedas, Tantra, and Kama Sutra. But, current social norms consider sex immoral. The high prevalence of porn consumption, child sexual abuse, child brides, and teenage pregnancies proves the need for sex education to be normalized.

Although Sakshi hasn't practiced in other countries, she has worked with people worldwide as clients and on projects with students and clinicians. She notes that Indians are not the only people who are sexually conservative. Many regions have the same concerns, values, sexual scripts, and unqualified professionals.

Certifications aren't required for specialties in India. There are no board certifications, so anyone can claim to be an expert. Elsewhere, interdisciplinary teams are valued and include occupational therapy. But in India, referrals are marked as "OT/PT," making no distinction between occupational therapy and physical therapy. As a result, there is more competition than collaboration between the two professions. Pay is also meager in India, so many therapists leave the country for more opportunities and higher pay. Most occupational therapists work in metropolitan cities to get the highest salary. However, that pay is not enough to afford to live in the city.

Sakshi lets out a long, loud laugh when I ask if the profession is representative of her culture. Treated like an outcast for talking about sexuality, she is pushed even further out when including children in these services. Her heritage is Hindu Kashmiri Pandit, an oppressed population in India with no home community because of religious persecution forcing them from their home region. In her years of school and practice, she has never met an occupational therapist who shares her heritage.

When attending global events, she finds herself explaining basic occupations and how they differ in India. For example, meals at home are often eaten on the floor sitting cross-legged; eating with hands is more common than using utensils; most people wear chappals (sandals) or go barefoot; bathtubs are for the elite; showers are only available to those who can afford them, a bucket of water with a mug is the most common way to take a shower; toilet tissue is not used; and latrines are more available than Western toilets. Indian culture is not monolithic. In fact, she has been spending more time learning about her own culture and religion. This has influenced her to consider religion in initial assessments and practice, prioritizing what is important to the person.

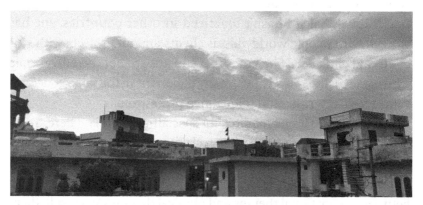

Figure 16.3: View from Sakshi's grandparents' home in Jammu

There are nuances to the many languages and cultures in the country. For instance, Sakshi knows at least ten ways to drape a sari, but there are even more ways to do it and different pleat styles on top of that. In some cultures and religions, when a person is menstruating, they cannot enter a temple or cook in the kitchen; while in others, these things are allowed. Though most Indians are fluent in English, many find terms like pronouns, gender, sex, and relationship styles confusing on Sakshi's intake forms, even though they are written in English. These are concepts that the average person is unfamiliar with.

"Everything we do, every single occupation, our existence, is political," she proclaims. The world we live in is based on hierarchy, and we are all oppressed and privileged in different parts of our life. Privilege affords greater access to healthcare and education, and in India, people from the higher castes are afforded more rights, privileges, and access. While those from the lower caste, Dalits, face greater discrimination, poverty, and mortality. India's caste system has been around for over 3000 years and dictates social and religious hierarchy, determining a person's place in society at birth. Although the practice of discrimination and segregation by caste was banned, the system is still in place, and caste distinctions are obvious.

Daily life issues in India, like abortion, pregnancy, and feminine hygiene, are political. Occupational therapy goes beyond activities of daily living, and her role is inherently political. An example is menstrual cups, reusable feminine hygiene products, in a country with sparse access to sanitary napkins. It seems like an easy and sustainable solution, but there are many people who, for reasons such as poverty, cannot use them. One cup costs 500 rupees, almost three times the daily minimum wage. A one-time investment can be cost-prohibitive and requires additional considerations like access to clean water, storage, and disinfectant soap. People who cannot afford to feed themselves cannot access these things.

If you've never watched a Bollywood movie or visited Mumbai, Sakshi describes it as the city of dreams and "beautiful madness." It's both beautiful and sad, filled with many stories in one crowded place. She lives in an air-conditioned apartment with nice furniture, delicious food, and anything she could need within reach. Through the window, she can see tents where people live with no running water, exposed to the elements and dangers of the city. Still, everyone has their role, and people come from all over the country to live in Mumbai.

Occupational therapy has been around in India for a long time. However, as the first program in Asia, it should be further ahead with recognition and involvement in interdisciplinary teams and specialties. Sakshi's hopes for occupational therapy in India include more practice areas that address mental health and sexuality—ideally, included in all settings. In addition, she wants the referral process to move past "OT/PT" to recognize occupational therapy as a distinct profession with various specializations.

Occupational therapy practice is unique in every region. We can always learn from each other in other parts of the world. She wants us to learn to be uncomfortable and step outside what we know. Connecting with the global occupational therapy community can help us understand more about practices, cultures, religions, and people. Social media makes it easy and free to access educational content worldwide.

Some of her recommendations to step out of our comfort zones are the *Man Enough* podcast, which attempts to redefine masculinity and gender roles; Hijabi OT on Instagram, a Bengali American hijabi occupational therapy student who shares information on cultural occupations; and free events from DisruptOT.

We all have unique experiences and preferences. Knowing everything is impossible, so we have to ask instead of assuming. Sakshi suggests removing the primary focus from diagnosis or illness to include the various identities of the people we work with, like their spirituality, culture, relationships, sexual expression, education, finances, and all the things that contribute to their life experiences. We should be educating ourselves regularly and demanding more from ourselves, professional organizations, and society.

SUGGESTED NEXT STEPS

Reflection: What does sexuality mean to you? How comfortable are you talking about sexuality with your family, peers, partner(s), colleagues, and patients? What are the limitations for you when discussing topics of sexuality?

These questions will help in forming a foundation of your values, opinions, and beliefs about sexuality and what you understand about yourself. This reflection is essential to know what you can do, can't do, and where you need to improve without superimposing your ideologies and judgment onto your clients.

Action: How will you tie sexuality into your practice with your current knowledge base? How can you expand your knowledge base? Sakshi recommends starting by working on yourself, reading more about the mind and body, and focusing on skills, not just theories. Who can you refer clients to or seek information from if they want to explore an area of sexuality that you are not knowledgeable about or experienced in?

References

Tickoo, S. (2022). *SexCare: A Self-Help Guide to Sexual Wellness.* BlueRose Publishers.

About the Author

Sheela Roy Ivlev is a Bengali American occupational therapist, a certified integrative mental health professional, and a consultant in San Francisco, California, the unceded ancestral homeland of the Ramaytush Ohlone people.

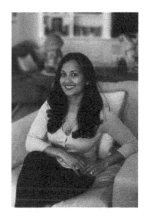

She is the founder of OT Bay Area, WellWrx Consulting, and DisruptOT, an international volunteer-based organization dedicated to disrupting the status quo in healthcare, challenging oppressive systems, building community, highlighting global voices, and providing free education to healthcare users, students, and practitioners worldwide.